Dr Sara's Honey Potions

By

Dr Sara Robb

For Helen

Best Wishes

Dr Sara Robb

Dr Sara's Honey Potions

By

Dr Sara Robb

Dedication
For Jesse and the Bug

Acknowledgements
Dr Sara would like to acknowledge Dr Sandip Patel and Chi Li for useful discussion.

Woodcuts
The Gardeners Kalendar by Philip Miller M.DCC.XXXIV
Gardener to the Worfhipful Company of Apothecaries
at their Botanick Garden in Chelfea

ISBN 978-1-904846-36-9

Northern Bee Books

Published 2009
Ruxbury Publications

Set in Gill Sans

Design and Artwork
D&P Design and Print
Redditch, Worcestershire

Measurement Equivalents
Units of Volume
1 tsp – teaspoon = 5 milliliters
1 T- tablespoon = 15 milliliters
¼ C – ¼ cup = 56 milliliters
½ C – ½ cup = 112.5 milliliters
1 C- cup = 225 milliliters
1 ml- milliliter = 1/5 teaspoon
5 ml- 5 milliliters = 1 teaspoon
10 ml- 10 milliliters = 2 teaspoons
15 ml- 15 milliliters = 3 teaspoons or 1 tablespoon

Units of Mass or Weight
1 mg- 1 milligram = 0.001 gram
1 g – 1 gram = 1000 milligrams
1 oz- 1 ounce = 28.35 grams
w/w % - weight to weight percentage = weight of solute/ (weight of solute + weight of solvent) * 100

Table of Contents

Preface

I grew up in Iowa, farm country of Midwest America. Most of the land is covered by fields of corn and soybeans and local people often have large vegetable gardens. Iowans have an appreciation of fresh produce and natural food products. In a typical Midwestern cupboard, you will find preserves, molasses and honey. I can picture my mother's cupboard and the large jar of honey kept there. The honey was a commercial honey made with the nectar of clover flowers. At the time I did not have an appreciation of how the bees collected the nectar or even where the honey came from. I just always expected it to be there when I opened the cupboard. My personal favourite use for honey was on a peanut butter sandwich. Chunky peanut butter was applied to a piece of bread in vast amounts and then drizzled with clover honey. The ratio of peanut butter to honey tended to vary with my mood but most often the honey ended up in the majority. I still make this delicacy today and still seem to end up sticky after making and eating a honey and peanut butter sandwich.

This is something I probably should not admit, but enjoying my peanut butter and honey sandwich was the extent of my appreciation of honey. Beekeepers, be advised, I have been converted and now have a much greater appreciation of the value of both honey and bees. My enlightenment was the result of a gift I received from my neighbour. She gave me a jar of Polish blossom honey. This jar of honey was unlike the honey I enjoyed in Iowa. It was crystalline and a much darker golden colour. At the time, I wondered what I would do with this honey. I cannot get my favourite peanut butter in the UK so my gourmet sandwich was not an option. I had been making soap for about a year so I thought I would make soap with the Polish blossom honey. Honey soap was something I had heard of but not something I had ever used and I certainly had no experience making honey soap. I do tend to try things and see what happens, so I gave it a go. I made my basic soap recipe of sunflower, coconut, palm and olive oil and added a large tablespoon of honey. The soap did not seem remarkably different when I stirred in the honey. However, as the soap started to thicken, the colour changed to a golden pumpkin colour. The soap mixture also had a sugary smell, similar to caramelised sugar blended with honey. I was very excited to try the finished soap. At least the honey soap would be interesting and I suspected it would be very nice. The soap had a yellow colour when it had set, much lighter than the golden pumpkin colour it had when I poured it into the pan. The fragrance continued to remind me of caramelised sugar. I was very eager to try the soap!

I have always been happy with my soap recipe; it lathers well and is very moisturizing and gentle. It is gentle enough that I began using my soap on my daughter Jasmine when she was six months old. By the time I made honey soap, Jasmine was 1½ years old. Miss

Jasmine was lucky enough to be the first to use my new honey soap. I ran a bath for Jasmine and in she went with a bar of golden honey soap. The soap lathered well and had a lovely smell. I was most impressed by how soft the soap was to the touch. I washed Jasmine with the experimental honey bar and must say when I took her out of the bath I was amazed by how soft her skin was. Jasmine felt as though she had applied lotion from head to toe. The addition of a spoonful of honey transformed the soap, giving it a remarkable moisturising quality which seemed disproportionate to the tiny amount of honey added to the soap recipe. This first honey soap served as an inspiration to me to make a number of honey toiletries and sparked an interest in both honey and bees.

A spoonful of honey added to my basic soap recipe has lead to the development of a number of honey soaps and other honey products. I have enjoyed experimenting with different types of honey in soaps. Jasmine also enjoys these experiments because she is the one who licks the spoon. As a result, Jasmine also has an interest in honey, bees and honey toiletries. Jasmine enjoys using honey bath bombs, beeswax lip balms, honey creams and honey soap. I have since had another daughter and have been using honey products on her from the time she was born. Meghan uses honey soap, as well as lavender and honey cream. My girls like to have a bath together with my lavender and honey foam bath. I continue to develop honey products and have been compiling my recipes through the years.

This book is a collection of my methods and recipes using honey and beeswax in toiletries. These recipes can be made with ingredients you can buy at the grocery store and do not require any special equipment. I hope you enjoy making and using honey toiletries and experimenting with your own honey.

Dr Sara

Chapter 1

Making Your Own Toiletries With Honey And Beeswax

The first thing to consider when you begin to make toiletries is what you would like to achieve. Are you making things for the enjoyment of creating or are you planning on giving the items as gifts? If you are experimenting and enjoy making things as an activity, it may not be important to package the toiletries. If you plan to give your products as gifts, you will want to consider how to present your beautiful handmade products.

You may want to make toiletries for your own use for specific reasons, such as having control of the ingredients. One advantage of making your own soaps and toiletries is that you control the ingredients. Perhaps you wish to avoid preservatives, animal fats or an allergen. Making your own products allows you to do so. Many commercially available-soaps contain animal fat, something that many people would rather not have in their cosmetics. So, one of the biggest advantages to making your own products is the control of ingredients.

I think a gift basket of honey toiletries you have made yourself is a wonderful present anyone would enjoy receiving. It is not just that these are things you have made yourself, but the quality of honey products is truly outstanding. Honey soaps, creams and potions have long been recognized for their moisturizing and healing properties. Both honey and beeswax add an emollient quality to cosmetics and toiletries and have been used for centuries in beauty treatments. Cleopatra is said to have washed with milk and honey. No doubt she had wonderfully soft skin. I have met a number of people who add a spoonful of honey to the bath to keep their skin soft and women who swear the application of honey to their face each night is the secret to looking young. While there are a few commercially available soaps and toiletries containing honey and beeswax, they are not available everywhere. Additionally, the beeswax used in cosmetics is very often refined, or had the colour and odour removed. I prefer products made with unrefined beeswax and enjoy experimenting with different kinds of honey in my products.

Making your own toiletries with honey and beeswax can be a very enjoyable hobby. You do not need any special equipment and can invest as much time and effort as you desire. An easy place to start is mixing honey into a product you buy at the shop. You can make interesting products using commercial products, such as creams, bubble baths, shampoo, or shower gel. Very often these products are already fragranced and so you can make a honey product with very little effort. In this case, little time or skill is needed. Adding honey to a favourite bubble bath is an easy activity for children and the resulting product can be put in a pretty bottle with a label made by the child. Even this simple mixing can be a fun activity and will build confidence to go on and try more difficult techniques. Why not add a little honey to your favourite bubble bath or shower gel?

Next, you might get a bit more adventurous and buy an unscented base product such as a cream or a lotion and add both honey and a fragrance. As you can image the combinations are endless at this level. You might add blossom honey and rose fragrance to a cream base for a rose garden cream, or lavender honey and lavender fragrance to a foam bath base to make a lavender foam bath. Adding honey and fragrance to base toiletries uses a little more imagination, and is a very easy way of making interesting and quality products without spending a lot of time. Starting with such simple techniques will give you a feel for adding honey to cosmetics and build your confidence. Making toiletries is very much like cooking. As you master the techniques, you become more skilled and are more easily able to succeed at recipes requiring more difficult methods. Stirring honey into a base product gives you an idea of how much honey to add and what the final product should feel like. This knowledge is useful when trying more difficult recipes.

After you have made toiletries with base products, many of you will want to make your own toiletries from scratch. The disadvantage of using base products is it is difficult to add beeswax to these products because the high melting temperature of beeswax will damage the product. By making toiletries from scratch you can add both the honey and the beeswax of your choice. Following a simple recipe, you can make your own lip balm with unrefined beeswax. I find lip balms made with unrefined beeswax to be much more pleasant to use and to have a pleasing beeswax aroma. Additionally, lovely soaps can be made incorporating honey and beeswax from the same hive. I think a basket with honey and beeswax soap and a jar of honey from the same hive would make a very nice present indeed.

Finally, some of you will go on to formulate your own recipes. Making toiletries such as soap with your own formulation can be very satisfying for those of you who like to experiment. Some of the beekeepers who have seen my soap making demonstration have gone on to formulate their own soap. Why not try adding other hive products such as propalis or royal jelly to your formulations? You are limited only by your imagination. As you can see, you can make your own honey products at any of these levels and will enjoy making and using the toiletries from your kitchen.

Chapter 2

The Use Of Colour In Toiletries

Unscented toiletries are like a blank canvass. The addition of colour and fragrance in various combinations unleashes creativity. The combinations are truly endless and allow you to make personalized potions for the special people in your life. For instance, by adding lavender essential oil and purple colour to a soap recipe, you will make a beautiful lavender coloured soap which will be very relaxing when used. If you make a pink bubble bath which smells like bubble gum, you can easily see this would be a fun product for a child to use. You can have a lot of fun combining different colours and fragrances and are only limited by your imagination.

The addition of colour to toiletries adds atheistic value to the products. It is appealing to colour honey soap a golden yellow or a lavender bath bomb a shade of purple. The colourant does not usually change the quality of the product however does make the product more pleasing to look at, and, as a result, use.

When adding colour to cosmetics and toiletries, one needs to consider both the product being coloured and the colouring substance. A basic understanding of the characteristics of the product you are making and the colour available will help you decide which colours are appropriate for which products and help to avoid disasters. For instance, if you are making a lip balm and try to add a water based colour to your lip balm base, you will end up with the colour separating from the lip balm. If however, you add an oil dispersible pigment, it will incorporate well into the product yielding a satisfactory result.

The chemicals used to add colour to toiletries and cosmetics are either organic or inorganic. Organic colours are of biological origin, while inorganic colours are not. Substances used to add colour can be further divided into water soluble colours and pigments. Water soluble colours are used to colour water based cosmetics such as bubble baths, shampoos and conditions. Pigments do not dissolve in the product being coloured but disperse in a suspension in the final product. These include both water based products such as bubble baths and oil based products such as lip balms. Pigment colours are very versatile and can be used to colour a wide range of products including soaps, bath bombs, and lip balms.

Table 1 lists some of the agents you can use to colour your cosmetics and toiletries. Substances used to add colour can be spices, organic pigments and inorganic pigments and water soluble dyes. Table 1 also gives additional information about some of the colours available, including the Colour Index number (CI number), the International Nomenclature for Cosmetic Ingredients (INCI) name, as well as recommended uses for each of the agents. The INCI name is used to label cosmetics. If you use a spice or botanical to change the hue of a product, then you will use the INCI name on the label. Agents that add colour seldom are listed by the INCI name, but rather the CI number. This number identifies agents used specifically as colourants. Each colouring agent is designated a specific number in the Colour Index. The Colour Index is published by The Society of Dyers and Colourist. Because spices and botanicals are not specifically colouring agents, they do not have CI numbers and would be listed by their INCI names.

Using spice to add colour is a traditional method of adding hue to products. Spices and botanicals do have many limitations. Beetroot powder is a beautiful purplish red and you might think would be a very good colourant to use in soap. This is not the case. The chemical which imparts the colour to beetroot actually looses its redness at high pH. I learned this the hard way. I added a heaped spoon of beetroot powder to a soap recipe and ended up with a pale yellow soap. Not at all the colour I was hoping for. Other drawbacks of using spices are that they may be irritating and add fragrance which may be undesirable. I do not think a cream or lip balm made with cayenne pepper would be very soothing. Finally, some spices and botanicals can stain. Beetroot and turmeric are good example. I am sure many of you have stained your countertops with beetroot and turmeric. One should consider these things when using spices and botanicals. Spices work well in soaps and a select few in other products.

Clays are another natural way to add colour to your products. I enjoy working with clay as it adds another dimension to the product. For instance adding French green clay to soap makes it more cleansing and yields a soap which is good for acne. French green clay does not have a CI number and as a result, is listed by its' INCI name, illite. Kaolin clay can also be used in soaps and toiletries. White kaolin has a CI number, CI 77004. There are other clays in a variety of colours which can add subtle tones to soaps, bath bombs and other products.

Pigments are colours which disperse through cosmetics and toiletries rather than dissolving. Because they disperse, pigments can be added to both water based and oil based products. I find pigments very interesting. Many of the pigments used to add colour to soap are the same pigments used in oil paints. If you are someone who paints with oil paints, you will recognise titanium white, ultramarine blue and other pigments listed in Table 1. Soapmakers use titanium dioxide to make soap white. Ultramarine blue and pink are frequently used in soaps as well. Additionally, chromium green oxide and the iron oxides are frequently listed as ingredients on cosmetic labels, and are all oxides used in oil paints. Titanium dioxide is very versatile and can be used in all the products listed including: soap, bath bombs, bubble bath creams and lip balms. Titanium white adds opacity to products. A little titanium dioxide goes a long way.

The ultramarines are also flexible colouring agents. Ultramarines are interesting in that the two colours, pink and blue, share the same CI number (CI 77007). A third shade, ultramarine purple is made by mixing ultramarine blue with ultramarine pink. In my experience, the ultramarine blue is very powerful and not much is needed. The ultramarine pink however, is much weaker and so much more is needed to colour the same volume. When I mix the blue and pink to make purple, I start with a large volume of pink and slowly and small quantities of blue until I reach a nice shade of purple. When I use ultramarine blue in soaps and other toiletries, I start with a tiny pinch and add until I like the colour. With both ultramarine pink and ultramarine purple, I tend to start with a spoonful to get the same effect as the pinch of blue gives. Ultramarines are frequently used in soaps, bath bombs, bubble baths, creams and lip balms. If you want to add a colour and are not sure where to start, I would try one of the ultramarines.

The iron oxides are pigments which come in a number of colours depending on the oxidation state of iron. I suppose iron oxides should be my favourite colours since I worked in an iron laboratory while researching for my PhD. In fact I studied how iron induces oxidative stress in neurodegenerative diseases. It is the chemical nature of iron oxides which enables them to come in a number of shades. Each colour of iron oxide has its own CI number. They add a lot of colour when a little is added and impart lovely earthy tones to toiletries such as soaps and lip balms. I do not use them in bath bombs because I worry about staining, similar to rust, another iron oxide. Addition of iron oxides to creams could also promote oxidative damage to the product so I tend to avoid adding iron oxides to creams. If you would like to add an iron oxide to cream products, adding the antioxidant, vitamin E may keep the oxidation in check.

Chromium green oxides are similar to the iron oxides but can be used in a broader range of products. Chromium oxide produces a beautiful mossy green in to soaps and other toiletries. Not much is needed. When I make a kilogram of soap, I add approximately ¼ teaspoon of chromium green oxide. Similarly, if you want to add colour to bubble bath or cream, I would begin with a tiny pinch and add sparingly until you get the desired colour.

Finally, manganese violet, the last metal-based pigment in the Table I is a brilliant violet colour unmatched by the other pigments. Unfortunately manganese oxide does not work well in water based products such as bubble baths and creams. Additionally, it reacts in cold processed soap and does not yield a violet colour but a gray-brown shade. However, manganese violet is gorgeous in lip balms. The colour is a lovely mauve. I was very impressed the first time I added manganese violet to a beeswax lip balm. Manganese violet and a little mica produce a lip balm colour any little girl would love. I use manganese violet in my Pink Lemonade lip balm and am always delighted with the colour.

The D&C colours and the FD&C colours are water based colours. For a long time I wondered what D&C and FD&C indicated. Now it seems so obvious. D&C colours are colours which are approved in the USA for use in drugs and cosmetics. FD&C colours (you have probably guessed) are colours approved in the USA for use in food, drugs and cosmetics. These synthetic colours give brilliant shades and are very good in cosmetics and toiletries. I have listed a number of these in Table I. D&C and FD&C colours very often come in an aqueous solution, making them inappropriate to use in lip balms. If you are able to obtain them in powdered form, you may be able to incorporated them into oil based products such as lip balms. These water soluble colours are excellent in bath bombs. I use them in a powdered concentrated form to add colour to my bath bombs but have also used them in the aqueous form. FD&C colours are many times the colours sold as food colouring. If you want to add a little colour to a water based product and do not have cosmetic colours available, you may be able to use food colouring.

Table 1 Adding Colours

Name	Hue	INCI	CI
Alkanet Root	Purple	Alkanna Tinctoria	
Beetroot Powder	Red	Beta Vulgaris Root Powder	
Cayenne Powder	Red	Capsicum Frutescens	
Paprika Powder	Red	Capsicum Annuum Fruit Powder	
Spirulina Powder	Green	Spirulina Maxima	
Cinnamon Powder	Brown	Cinnamomum Cassia Bark	
Tumeric Powder	Yellow	Curcuma Longa Root Powder	
French Green Clay	Green	Illite	
Kaolin Clay	White	Kaolin	CI 7700
Titanium Dioxide	White	Titanium Dioxide	CI 7789
Yellow Iron Oxide	Yellow	CI 77492	CI 7749
Red Iron Oxide	Red	CI 77491	CI 7749
Brown Iron Oxide	Orange	CI 77489	CI 7748
Black Iron Oxide	Black	CI 77499	CI 7749
Ultramarine Pink	Pink	Ultramarines	CI 7700
Ultramarine Purple	Purple	Ultramarines	CI 7700
Ultramarine Blue	Blue	Ultramarines	CI 7700
Magnesium Violet	Violet	CI 77742	CI 7774
Chromium Green Oxide	Green	Chromium Oxide Greens	CI 7728
FD&C Blue No. 1	Blue	Blue 1 Lake	CI 4209
D&C Blue No. 4	Blue	Blue 1 Lake	CI 4209
D&C Red No. 7	Red	CI 15850	CI 1585
FD&C Red No. 33	Red	Acid Red 33	CI 1720
FD&C Yellow No. 6	Yellow	Sunset Yellow	CI 1598
FD&C Yellow No. 5	Yellow	Acid Yellow 23	CI 1914
D&C Yellow No. 10	Yellow	Acid Yellow 3 Aluminum Lake	CI 4700

INCI- International Nomenclature of Cosmetic Ingredie

Table 1 should be used a guide to help you add colour to your soaps and toiletries. It is not meant to be adhered to rigidly. Experiment. If you are happy with your results, that is what is most important. Table 1 is meant to give you a starting point and a little guidance in selecting colours to use in your potions.

Soap-CP	Bath Bombs	Bubble Bath	Cream	Lip Balm
X	X			X
				X
X				
X				
X				
X	X			
X				
X	X			
X	X			X
X	X	X	X	X
X				X
X				X
X				X
X				X
X	X	X	X	X
X	X	X	X	X
X	X	X	X	X
	X			X
X		X	X	
X	X	X	X	
X	X	X	X	
X	X	X	X	
X	X	X	X	
X	X	X	X	
X	X	X	X	
X	X	X	X	

Chemical Index Number, Soap **CP**- Cold Processed Soap

Chapter 3

The Use Of Fragrance In Toiletries

Just as adding colour to cosmetics adds a visual quality to your products, fragrance adds the further dimension of scent. There are an abundance of fragrance products available. Fragrances can be added in the form of fragrance oil or essential oil. Essential oils are natural scents derived from plants while fragrance oils can be in part natural or completely synthesised. Some fragrances are synthesized because the essential oil is very pricey. One of my favourite laboratory exercises as a student was in organic chemistry, where we synthesized jasmine fragrance. Natural jasmine is very expensive and the synthesized fragrance is much less expensive. It can be very enjoyable to combine various fragrances with colours in toiletries. By combining different colours and fragrances, you create your own unique products. I like to think about who I am making the toiletries for and then combine colours and fragrances I think the person will like. For instance, for my daughter Jasmine, I made a line of products in sugar plum fragrance, using honey and in pink (obviously). Jasmine is the original Sugar Plum Girl!

Before you begin, it is important to consider who you are making your potions for and whether you will use essential oils or fragrance oils. Essential oils and fragrance oils differ in a number of ways. Essential oils are composed of the natural chemicals isolated from a specific plant. Fragrance oils are composed of chemicals either isolated from natural products or synthesized. Essential oils are sometimes more true to the aroma of the plant, however many fragrance oils are also true to the smell of plants. Fragrance oils offer a larger variety of fragrances because some of them are made to smell like things other than plants. For instance, you can get fragrance oils in bubble gum, honey or even like your favourite perfume.

Both essential oils and fragrance oils can be irritating to the skin. You can limit the irritation by making unscented products, decreasing the fragrance in the product or using fragrances which are less irritating. In my experience, essential oils are more irritating than fragrance oils in the same fragrance. I have made soap with lavender essential oil, which I found irritating, and lavender fragrance oil, which I did not find irritating. Others may find the reverse. Additionally, I find citrus fragrances to be quite irritating in both essential oils and fragrance oils. I tend to avoid citrus fragrance if I know someone has sensitive skin. I like the smell of citrus but cannot use products fragranced with citrus fragrance unless honey is added to the product as well. In my experience, the addition of honey also makes products less irritating to the skin.

Another difference between essential oils and fragrance oils is that fragrance oils are not used medically, while essential oils can be bioactive and used medicinally. Because essential oils can have bioactivity, there are a number of contraindications for essential oils, while fragrance oils tend to be safe for most users. The following essentials oils should never be used neat on the skin; alan root, bitter almond, bergamot, sweet birch, birch tar, boldo leaf, cade, calamus, camphor, cassis, cinnamon bark, colophon, costus root, fig leaf, horseradish, mustard, opoponax, peru balsam, rue, sassafras, tansy, tolu, turpentine, verbena, and wintergreen. It is recommended these be diluted into a carrier oil if they are to be used on the skin.

Essential oils in general are not considered safe for children. And many essential oils are not considered safe for pregnant and breastfeeding women. Women who are pregnant or breastfeeding should avoid products made with; basil, cedar wood, clary sage, fennel, jasmine, lavender, marjoram, myrrh, rose, rosemary, sage and thyme. Remember that essential oils are very concentrated and contain much greater quantities of the bioactive chemicals than same weight of the plant themselves. So while it may be safe to eat many on the aforementioned list in food, it is not safe to use the essential oils in products when you are pregnant or breastfeeding. Finally, many essential oils are contraindicated for epileptics. People suffering from epilepsy should not use product containing: cajaput, camphor, eucalyptus, fennel, hyssop, peppermint, and rosemary. If you choose to use essential oil, make sure you consider who will use the products and consider the contraindications.

The amount of fragrance you use in each product will depend on the intended use of the product. In general, if a toiletry will be applied directly to the skin and not washed away, you will want to add a smaller amount of fragrance. If a product will be diluted into the bath, a higher concentration of fragrance should be used. So less fragrance is used in creams than in bath oils. Table 2 is a guide to how much fragrance to add to your honey potions. The quantities should be used as a guideline. You may find there will be situations where you will want to increase the fragrance slightly or decrease it slightly. I find some fragrances work better at lower concentrations and so decrease the amount I add. For instance, jasmine and rose fragrance oils both give strong fragrance to products so I add less of those to my products.

Table 2

Guide for Adding fragrance

Product	Light	Medium	Strong
Soap	2% w/w	3% w/w	5% w/w
Bath Oil	5% w/w	10% w/w	15% w/w
Bubble Bath	5% w/w	7% w/w	10% w/w
Bath Bombs	1 % w/w	5 % w/w	10% w/w
Lotions/Creams/ Massage Oil	0.5% w/w	1% w/w	2.5%w/w
Shower Gel/ Shampoo/Conditioner	2% w/w	3% w/w	5% w/w

Table 2 shows suggested amounts of fragrance to add to different toiletries. The amounts are listed as a percentage of weight to weight calculated as "weight of the solute/ (weight of solute + weight of solvent) x 100". When making your own products use the quantity in the "light" column if you would like make a product with less fragrance or when making something for someone with sensitive skin. The "medium" column will give products with a moderate amount of fragrance which will be enjoyed while the product is being used, yet will only leave a subtle fragrance on the skin. Higher amounts of fragrance can be used, such as indicated in the "strong" column. Toiletries made with higher concentrations of fragrances will likely leave fragrance on the skin and will be appreciated by those who prefer stronger scented products. In summary, it is all a matter of taste and skin type.

Chapter 4

Adding Honey To Cosmetic Base Products

Working with base products is a good place to start when you begin to make toiletries. Base products are commercially available form a number of suppliers. All you need to do is add a little fragrance, honey and perhaps some colour to have a unique product you have made yourself. However if you would like to make something with minimal investment, get a bottle of fragranced bubble bath form the supermarket and add some honey to that. Children love to mix things and will feel a great sense of satisfaction after adding honey to a bubble bath and putting it into a pretty bottle. Add a label that says "handmade for you by" I am sure you will find this activity is met with a mass of enthusiasm.

Unscented base products enable you to combine a variety of fragrances, colours and different types of honey. In my shop we use base products at our Potion Parties. Unscented base products are incredibly versatile. The same base can become Pink Lemonade Bubble Bath at one party and Honey Bee Bubble Bath at another, simply by changing the fragrance and honey added to the base and the label applied to the bottle.

When adding honey to base toiletries, less should be used in products that will be left on the skin, such as creams and lotions. If the product will be washed away, more honey can be added, for instance in face masks, scrubs and soaps. Additionally, more honey can be added to products like bubble bath which will be diluted when added to the bath. It does not take much honey to transform a nice toiletry into an outstanding toiletry.

Another consideration is the kind of honey used. If the honey is crystalline, you may wish to melt it to dissolve the sugar crystals before adding to a cream or lotion. If making a sugar scrub with honey, the crystals may add to the exfoliating quality of the scrub. It is likely that if you do not melt the crystals, they will eventually dissolve in the cosmetic base as most are water based. Taking the time to dissolve the crystals will make mixing the honey into the product easier.

I am sure you have noticed I have not mentioned adding beeswax to base cosmetics. It is difficult to add beeswax to base toiletries due to the high melting temperature of the beeswax. In order to add beeswax to a cream, you would need to significantly heat the base cream and this could lead to the cream separating. Beeswax is best added when the cosmetic is initially made. Additionally, many of the base products used to make toiletries are water based and beeswax is not water soluble. Similarly, when working with Lip balm base, which is oil based, honey will be difficult to add due to it's inability to combine with oil.

Table 3

Guidelines For Adding Honey To Base Products

Product	Honey
Soap	3% w/w
Bubble Bath	5% w/w
Bath Bombs	1% w/w
Lotions/Creams	1% w/w
Shower Gel/Shampoo/Conditioner	2.5% w/w

The amounts suggested in Table 3 are appropriate when adding honey to toiletries which already contain fragrance, adding honey to unscented base products, and also when making toiletries from scratch. The same recommendations apply when adding honey to products as when adding fragrance. If you are making a product which will stay on the skin and not be washed away, such as a cream, you should use a smaller amount of honey to avoid stickiness. When making foam baths with honey, a higher amount of honey can be used because it will be diluted into a large volume of water in the bath. Soap is also washed away so, although it is used directly on the skin, it will be rinsed away so you have a lot of flexibility in how much honey you can add.

Following are a few suggested recipes beginning with the most basic, adding honey to a fragranced bubble bath.

Very Easy Honey Bee Bubble Bath

Ingredients
1/2 C Bubble bath*
1 tsp Honey

Equipment
A measuring cup or small coffee cup
Small bowl
Teaspoon
Funnel
Plastic bottle
Sticky label

*You can buy large bottles of inexpensive bubble bath at the supermarket. This bubble bath works well as a base for this children's recipe.

Making the Bubble Bath
1. Pour 1/2 C of bubble bath into the measuring cup or coffee cup.
2. Transfer the bubble bath to the small bowl.
3. Measure 1 tsp of your favourite honey on the teaspoon.
4. Mix the honey into the bubble bath. Stir until all the honey has been mixed through.
5. Use the funnel to put the bubble bath into the plastic bottle.
6. Design a label for your Honey Bee Bubble Bath. Maybe add "Handmade by" and your name.

Lavender Honey Cream

Ingredients	*Equipment*
100 g / 3.5 oz Base cream	Scale
1 ml / small drop Lavender honey	Teaspoon
1 ml / small drop Lavender fragrance oil	Small bowl
	100 ml Plastic jar

*You can substitute a variety of fragrances and honey to create a number of different creams

Making the Cream
1. Put the bowl on the scale and zero.
2. Weigh 100 g / 3.5 oz base moisture cream into the small bowl.
3. Add 1 ml / small drop Lavender honey to the bowl containing the cream.
4. Add 1 ml/ small drop Lavender fragrance to the bowl containing the cream and honey.
5. Mix thoroughly to incorporate the honey and fragrance into the cream.
6. Transfer the cream to the cream jar .

Orange Blossom Bubble Bath

Ingredients	*Equipment*
125 g / 4.4 oz Bubble bath base	Scale
5ml/ 1 tsp Blossom honey*	Small bowl
5 ml /1 tsp Orange fragrance oil*	Teaspoon
	Mixing spoon
	Funnel
	Plastic bottle

*You can use any fragrance oil and honey combination in this recipe

Making the Bubble Bath
1. Place the bowl on the scale and tare out the weight.
2. Weigh 125g / 4.4 oz base bubble bath into bowl.
3. Measure 5ml/ 1 tsp of your blossom honey and put in bowl containing the bubble bath base.
4. Measure 5ml/ 1 tsp orange fragrance oil and add to the bowl containing the bubble bath and honey.
5. Mix the honey and fragrance oil into the bubble bath.
6. Use the funnel to put the bubble bath into the plastic bottle.

Sunny Honey Lotion

Ingredients	*Equipment*
100 g / 3.5 oz Base lotion	Scale
1 ml/ small drop Sunflower honey*	Small bowl
1 ml/ small drop Sunflower fragrance oil*	Teaspoon
	Mixing spoon
	Funnel
	Plastic bottle

*You can substitute a variety of fragrances and honey to create a number of different creams

Making the Lotion
1. Place the bowl on the scale and tare out the weight.
2. Weigh 100 g / 3.5 oz base bubble bath into bowl.
3. Measure 1 ml/ 1 small drop of your sunflower honey and put in bowl containing the bubble bath base.
4. Measure 1 ml/ 1 small drop sunflower fragrance oil and add to the bowl containing the bubble bath and honey.
5. Mix the honey and fragrance oil into the bubble bath.
6. Use the funnel to put the bubble bath into the plastic bottle.

Chapter 5

Dr Sara's Honey Bath Bombs

Making bath bombs can be enjoyed by the whole family. I find children are very impressed when they see the bombs they have made fizz when put into water. Bath bombs are relatively easy to make and can be made with readily available ingredients and utensils you have in your kitchen. Old and young alike will enjoy doing a bit of "kitchen chemistry" and seeing the bombs fizz. The ingredients you will need are citric acid and sodium bicarbonate. These are the chemicals that react when placed in water to generate the fizz. The sodium bicarbonate and citric acid react to produce carbon dioxide gas, the same gas in fizzy pop. Sodium bicarbonate is the white powder used in baking and is non-irritating. Citric acid, is the acid found in citric fruit and is an irritant. If you have ever got lemon juice into a cut, you will know this stings and citric acid does the same. Because of this, you will want to ensure that any children making bombs wear gloves and are careful with the powder. Kitchen gloves are fine and afford enough protection. However, if you really want to look the part of the kitchen chemist, laboratory gloves will do the trick. Maybe you have used bath bombs in the past and found them irritating to the skin. Adding honey to bath bombs decreases this irritation. I have found the Honey & Carrot Bee Bombs gentle enough for Meghan to use.

You will also want to add some fragrance to your bath bombs and perhaps some colour. You can use food colouring. This is the simplest form of colour for making bath bombs. Remember many of the colours used to make bath bombs are the same as those in food colours (the FD&C colours- see Table 1) Alternatively, you can by concentrated aqueous and powdered colours sold as cosmetic colours. Because the cosmetic colours are very concentrated, they should be used sparingly. The addition of too much of these agents can lead to staining of plastic baths and fabrics. The cosmetic colours sold for making bath bombs are available in a variety of colours and yield very pretty bath bombs. The colour you choose to make your bath bombs might match the fragrance you use. For instance, you might like to make lavender bath bombs a light purple colour.

The fragrance you use to add scent to your honey bath bombs should be oil based, for instance, a fragrance oil or essential oil. If you want to use a fragrance that is water or alcohol based, you will need to decrease to amount of water in the recipe. Perhaps you would like to make bath bombs and do not have any fragrance oil but have some vanilla extract in the kitchen. You could use vanilla extract, but remember this will count as some of your water. If you add too much water, it is not the end of the world. The bombs will swell and be like puffy marshmallows. They may not give as much fizz when you put them in the bath but you will enjoy them just the same.

Bath bomb recipes are based on the chemical reaction of the citric acid with the bicarbonate. Three sodium bicarbonate molecules react with one citric acid molecule to produce three molecules of carbon dioxide gas. Bath bomb recipes take this chemical reaction into account. A good bath bomb recipe will have the correct ratio of sodium bicarbonate to citric acid. However, three molecules of sodium bicarbonate to one molecule of citric acid does not work out to three times the volume or even weight of sodium bicarbonate to citric acid. Because the molecules have different weights, the ratio is actually two times the weight of sodium bicarbonate to one part of citric acid. The recipes herein are based on the actual chemical reaction and take into account the weight of the molecules. This gives you the correct ratio and leads to very fizzy bath bombs. Having pointed this out, if you get the ratio slightly wrong, it will not completely ruin the bombs or even make a dangerous product. Many recipes call for three times the weight or volume of sodium bicarbonate to citric acid, this will result in an excess of sodium bicarbonate. If you use a recipe which calls for three times sodium bicarbonate, you will just have too much bicarbonate. Having an excess of sodium bicarbonate just means there will be bicarbonate molecules, which will not have citric acid molecules to react with. Because getting it slightly wrong does not matter that much, you can measure the ingredients by volume or weight and still produce a very nice finished product.

The equipment you will need is as follows; a large bowl, a smaller bowl or cup, gloves, moulds, measuring spoons and scales. You really can use almost anything for a mould. I have used chocolate moulds, ice cube trays, soap moulds and moulds designed to make bath bombs. If you find the shape interesting, why not give it a try. Remember if you are adding fragrance and use plastic bowls and moulds, the plastic will retain some of the fragrance. You may wish to dedicate these for use in bath bomb making. Alternatively, you can use a glass bowl to mix the bombs, the moulds however are almost all plastic and so should be specifically for use with fragrances (making soaps, bath bombs, etc.).

Very Easy Bath Bombs

Ingredients
1 C Sodium bicarbonate
½ C Citric acid
½ tsp Honey
1 tsp Food colouring
1 tsp Fragrance
1 tsp Vegetable oil

Equipment
A measuring cup or small coffee cup
Teaspoon
Large bowl
Small bowl
Ice cube tray
Gloves
Greaseproof paper

Making the Bath Bombs

1. Wearing your gloves, measure 1 C of sodium bicarbonate and place into large bowl

2. Measure ½ C of citric acid and place in large bowl containing the sodium bicarbonate.

3. Mix the sodium bicarbonate and citric acid with your hands. Break up any lumps as you mix.

4. Into a small bowl measure the liquid ingredients: 1 tsp food colouring, 1 tsp vegetable oil, ½ tsp honey, and 1 tsp fragrance.

5. Mix the liquid ingredients well. The oil and water will not stay mixed.

6. Add the liquid ingredients to your dry mixture of sodium bicarbonate and citric acid. When you add the liquid, you will see a little fizzing. This is because the sodium bicarbonate is reacting with the citric acid to produce carbon dioxide.

7. Using your hands, mix the liquid into the dry ingredients. You will know when you have mixed well because the colour will become uniform and there will be no dry areas.

8. Begin to fill your ice cube tray with the bath bomb mixture. Press the powder in firmly to ensure the shape holds together.

9. After all the cavities have been filled, turn the bath bombs out onto some greaseproof paper.

10. Allow the bath bombs to dry

Honey & Carrot Bee Bombs

Ingredients	Equipment
800 g / 28 oz Sodium bicarbonate	A scoop
400 g / 14 oz Citric acid	Weighing scales
10 ml / 2 tsp Honey	Measuring spoons
15 ml / 3 tsp Water	Sieve
10 ml / 2 tsp Fragrance of your choice such	Large bowl
as sunflower or orange	Small bowl
10 ml / 2 tsp Carrot oil	Bee moulds
	Gloves
	Greaseproof paper

Making the Bath Bombs

1. Place your large bowl on the scales. Place the sieve on top of the bowl and zero the scale.

2. Wearing your gloves, scoop 800 g / 28 oz sodium bicarbonate into the sieve and sieve into the large bowl.

3. Zero the scale again. Scoop 400 g / 14 oz of citric acid into the sieve. Sift the citric acid into the large bowl containing the sodium bicarbonate.

4. Mix the sodium bicarbonate and citric acid with your hands.
5. Into a small bowl measure the liquid ingredients: 15 ml / 3tsp water, 10 ml / 2 tsp carrot oil, 10 ml / 2 tsp honey, and 10 ml / 2 tsp fragrance.
6. Mix the liquid ingredients well. The oil and water will not stay mixed.
7. Add the liquid ingredients to your dry mixture of sodium bicarbonate and citric acid. When you add the liquid, you will see a little fizzing. This is because the sodium bicarbonate is reacting with the citric acid to produce carbon dioxide.
8. Using your hands, mix the liquid into the dry ingredients. You will know when you have mixed well because the colour will become uniform and there will be no dry areas. The carrot oil will give the mixture a lovely yellow colour.
9. Begin to fill your bee moulds with the bath bomb mixture. Press the powder in firmly to ensure the shape holds together.
10. After all the cavities have been filled, turn the bath bombs out onto some greaseproof paper.
11. Allow the bath bombs to dry

Lavender Chamomile Honey Heart Bombs

Ingredients	Equipment
800 g / 28 oz Sodium bicarbonate	A scoop
400 g / 14 oz Citric acid	Weighing scales
10 ml / 2 tsp Lavender honey	Measuring spoons
15 ml / 3 tsp Water	Sieve
10 ml / 2 tsp Lavender fragrance oil	Large bowl
or essential oil	Small bowl
10 ml / 2 tsp Sunflower oil	Heart shaped moulds
1 sachet / 1 T Chamomile tea	Gloves
1 pinch Dry colour red (CI 15850;	Greaseproof paper
D&C Red No. 7)*	
1 pinch Ultramarine blue (CI 77007)*	

Making the Bath Bombs
1. Place the sieve on top of the bowl, put the bowl on the scale and zero.
2. Wearing your gloves, scoop 800 g / 28 oz sodium bicarbonate into the sieve and sieve into the large bowl
3. Zero the scale again. Scoop 400 g / 14 oz of citric acid into the sieve. Sift the citric acid into the large bowl containing the sodium bicarbonate.
4. Tear the chamomile tea bag open and add the chamomile flowers to the dry ingredients.
5. Add a pinch of the red pigment and the ultramarine blue to the dry ingredients.

6. Using your hands, blend the dry ingredients until the colour becomes uniform. You can adjust the colour to the shade of lavender you would like by adding slightly more red or blue pigment.
7. Into a small bowl measure the liquid ingredients: 15 ml / 3 tsp water, 10 ml / 2 tsp sunflower oil, 10 ml / 2 tsp lavender honey, and 10 ml / 2 tsp lavender fragrance.
8. Mix the liquid ingredients well. The oil and water will not stay mixed.
9. Add the liquid ingredients to your dry mixture. When you add the liquid, you will see a little fizzing. This is because the sodium bicarbonate is reacting with the citric acid to produce carbon dioxide.
10. Using your hands, mix the liquid into the dry ingredients. Mix well to distribute the liquid through the dry ingredients.
11. Begin to fill the heart moulds with the bath bomb mixture. Press the powder in firmly to ensure the shape holds together.
12. After all the cavities have been filled, turn the bath bombs out onto greaseproof paper.
13. Allow the bath bombs to dry

*if you do not have access to these cosmetic colours, you may substitute food colouring. Decrease the amount of water by the volume of food colouring added

Champagne & Honey Bath Bombs

Ingredients	Equipment
800 g / 28 oz Sodium bicarbonate	A scoop
400 g / 14 oz Citric acid	Weighing scales
10 ml / 2 tsp Blossom honey	Measuring spoons
15 ml / 3 tsp Champagne	Sieve
10 ml / 2 tsp Champagne fragrance oil	Large bowl
10 ml / 2 tsp Sunflower oil*	Small bowl
1 pinch Yellow iron oxide (CI 77492)	2" Heart moulds
1 tsp Mica powder	Gloves
	Greaseproof paper
	Small glass jar (approximately 20 ml volume works well)
	Small flower stamp
	Small plate

Making the stamping mica
1. Place 1 tsp mica power into a small glass jar.
2. Add a pinch of yellow iron oxide to the glass jar containing the mica.
3. Place the lid on the jar firmly and shake the jar to mix the mica and iron oxide.

4.   place a small amount of the gold mica powder on a small plate to use as a stamping pad.

Making the Bath Bombs

1.   Place your large bowl on the scales. Place the sieve on top of the bowl and zero the scale.
2.   Wearing your gloves, scoop 800 g / 28 oz sodium bicarbonate into the sieve and sieve into the large bowl
3.   Zero the scale again. Scoop 400 g / 14 oz of citric acid into the sieve. Sift the citric acid into the large bowl containing the sodium bicarbonate.
4.   Mix the sodium bicarbonate and citric acid with your hands.
5.   Into a small bowl measure the liquid ingredients: 15 ml / 3 tsp champagne, 10 ml / 2 tsp sunflower oil, 10 ml / 2 tsp blossom honey, and 10 ml / 2 tsp champagne fragrance.
6.   Mix the liquid ingredients well. The oil and champagne will not stay mixed so mix just prior to step 7.
7.   Add the liquid ingredients to your dry mixture of sodium bicarbonate and citric acid. When you add the liquid, you will see a little fizzing. This is because the sodium bicarbonate is reacting with the citric acid to produce carbon dioxide.
8.   Using your hands, mix the liquid into the dry ingredients. Mix well as there is no colouring agent to help you know when it is mixed. When you have mixed the ingredients well there will be no dry areas.
9.   Begin to fill the heart moulds with the bath bomb mixture. Press the powder in firmly into each cavity to ensure the shape holds together.
10. After all the cavities have been filled, turn the bath bombs out onto some greaseproof paper.
11. Press your flower stamp into the gold mica. Tap it into the mica a number of times to cover the stamp well. Tap again out of the mica to remove any excess mica. Stamp a gold mica flower onto each heart bomb. The gold flower adds a special touch to these champagne bombs.

*if you have a sunflower oil allergy, try soy oil as a substitute.

Pink Lemonade Bath Bombs

Ingredients
800 g / 28 oz Sodium bicarbonate
400 g / 14 oz Citric acid
10 ml / 2 tsp Heather honey
15 ml / 3 tsp Red food colouring
10 ml / 2 tsp Lemon fragrance
10 ml / 2 tsp Vegetable oil

Equipment
A scoop
Weighing scales
Measuring spoons
Sieve
Large bowl
Small bowl
Ice cube tray
Gloves
Greaseproof paper

Making the Bath Bombs

1. Place your large bowl on the scales. Place the sieve on top of the bowl and zero the scale.
2. Wearing your gloves, scoop 800 g / 28 oz sodium bicarbonate into the sieve and sieve into the large bowl
3. Zero the scale again. Scoop 400 g / 14 oz of citric acid into the sieve. Sift the citric acid into the large bowl containing the sodium bicarbonate.
4. Mix the sodium bicarbonate and citric acid with your hands.
5. Into a small bowl measure the liquid ingredients: 15 ml / 3 tsp red food colouring, 10 ml / 2 tsp vegetable oil, 10 ml / 2 tsp blossom honey, and 10 ml / 2 tsp lemon fragrance.
6. Mix the liquid ingredients well. The oil and water will not stay mixed.
7. Add the liquid ingredients to your dry mixture of sodium bicarbonate and citric acid. When you add the liquid, you will see a little fizzing. This is because the sodium bicarbonate is reacting with the citric acid to produce carbon dioxide.
8. Using your hands, mix the liquid into the dry ingredients. You will know when you have mixed well because the pink colour will become uniform and there will be no dry areas.
9. Begin to fill the ice cube tray with the bath bomb mixture. Press the powder in firmly to ensure the shape holds together.
10. After all the cavities have been filled, turn the bath bombs out onto some greaseproof paper.
11. Allow the bath bombs to dry

Pink Lemonade bath bombs are a favourite at Potion Parties. The girls like to make these in various shapes, including hearts, flowers, butterflies and ladybugs.

Rose Hip & Honey Bombs

Ingredients	Equipment
800 g / 28 oz Sodium bicarbonate	A scoop
400 g / 14 oz Citric acid	Weighing scales
10 ml / 2 tsp Blossom honey	Measuring spoons
10 ml / 2 tsp Rose water	Sieve
5 ml / 1 tsp Red food colouring	Large bowl
10 ml / 2 tsp Rose fragrance or essential oil	Small bowl
10 ml / 2 tsp Sweet almond oil*	Flower moulds
1 sachet of Rose hip tea	Gloves
	Greaseproof paper

Making the Bath Bombs

1. Place your large bowl on the scales. Place the sieve on top of the bowl and zero the scale.
2. Wearing your gloves, scoop 800 g / 28 oz sodium bicarbonate into the sieve and sieve into the large bowl
3. Zero the scale again. Scoop 400 g / 14 oz of citric acid into the sieve. Sift the citric acid into the large bowl containing the sodium bicarbonate.
4. Open the sachet of rose hip tea and empty the contents into the large bowl of bicarbonate and citric acid.
5. Mix the sodium bicarbonate, citric acid, and rose hip tea with your hands.
6. Into a small bowl measure the liquid ingredients: 10 ml / 2 tsp rose water, 5ml / 1 tsp red food colouring, 10 ml / 2 tsp sweet almond oil, 10 ml / 2 tsp blossom honey, and 10 ml / 2 tsp rose fragrance or essential oil.
7. Mix the liquid ingredients well. The oil and water will not stay mixed.
8. Add the liquid ingredients to your dry mixture of sodium bicarbonate and citric acid. When you add the liquid, you will see a little fizzing. This is because the sodium bicarbonate is reacting with the citric acid to produce carbon dioxide.
9. Using your hands, mix the liquid into the dry ingredients. You will know when you have mixed well because the colour will become uniform and there will be no dry areas. The bath bomb mixture will be a pale pink colour with darker specks of rose hip.
10. Begin to fill your flower moulds with the bath bomb mixture. Press the powder in firmly to ensure the shape holds together.
11. After all the cavities have been filled, turn the bath bombs out onto some greaseproof paper.
12. Allow the bath bombs to dry

*If you are concerned about nut allergies, you may substitute sunflower or vegetable oil for sweet almond oil.

Pink Champagne & Honey Hearts

Ingredients	Equipment
Ingredients	*Equipment*
800 g / 28 oz Sodium bicarbonate	A scoop
400 g / 14 oz Citric acid	Weighing scales
5 ml / 1 tsp Blossom honey	Measuring spoons
15 ml / 3 tsp Pink champagne	Sieve
5 ml / 1 tsp Rose Fragrance oil	Large bowl
5 ml / 1 tsp Champagne fragrance oil	Small bowl
10 ml / 2 tsp Sunflower oil	Miniature heart moulds
1 pinch Dry Red colour (CI 15850; D&C Red No. 7)	Gloves
1/8 tsp Mica	Greaseproof paper

Making the Bath Bombs

1. Place your large bowl on the scales. Place the sieve on top of the bowl and zero the scale.
2. Wearing your gloves, scoop 800 g / 28 oz sodium bicarbonate into the sieve and sieve into the large bowl
3. Zero the scale again. Scoop 400 g / 14 oz of citric acid into the sieve. Sift the citric acid into the large bowl containing the sodium bicarbonate.
4. Add a pinch of the red colour pigment and 1/8 teaspoon mica to the bicarbonate and citric acid.
5. Mix the sodium bicarbonate and citric acid with your hands until the powders are mixed evenly.
6. Into a small bowl measure the liquid ingredients: 15 ml / 3 tsp pink champagne, 5 ml / 1 tsp blossom honey, 5 ml / 1 tsp rose fragrance oil, 5 ml / 1 tsp champagne fragrance oil, and 10 ml / 2 tsp sunflower oil.
7. Mix the liquid ingredients well. The oil and champagne will not stay mixed so mix just prior to step 8.
8. Add the liquid ingredients to your dry mixture of sodium bicarbonate and citric acid. When you add the liquid, you will see a little fizzing. This is because the sodium bicarbonate is reacting with the citric acid to produce carbon dioxide.
9. Using your hands, mix the liquid into the dry ingredients. When you have mixed the ingredients well there will be no dry areas and the coour will be even.
10. Begin to fill the flower moulds with the bath bomb mixture. Press the powder in firmly into each cavity to ensure the shape holds together.
11. After all the cavities have been filled, turn the bath bombs out onto some greaseproof paper.

These tiny pink hearts look very nice in small boxes and make lovely wedding favours. Or put a few in a small organza bag as a special little gift.

Sunny Honey Bath Bombs

Ingredients
800 g / 28 oz Sodium bicarbonate
400 g / 14 oz Citric acid
10 ml / 2 tsp Sunflower honey
15 ml / 3 tsp Yellow food colouring
10 ml / 2 tsp Sunflower fragrance oil
10 ml / 2 tsp Sunflower oil

Equipment
A scoop
Weighing scales
Measuring spoons
Sieve
Large bowl
Small bowl
Flower moulds
Gloves
Greaseproof paper

Making the Bath Bombs

1. Place your large bowl on the scales. Place the sieve on top of the bowl and zero the scale.
2. Wearing your gloves, scoop 800 g / 28 oz sodium bicarbonate into the sieve and sieve into the large bowl
3. Zero the scale again. Scoop 400 g / 14 oz of citric acid into the sieve. Sift the citric acid into the large bowl containing the sodium bicarbonate.
4. Mix the sodium bicarbonate, and citric acid, with your hands until the powders are mixed evenly.
5. Into a small bowl measure the liquid ingredients: 15 ml / 3 tsp yellow food colouring, 10 ml / 2 tsp sunflower oil, 10 ml / 2 tsp sunflower honey, and 5 ml / 1 tsp sunflower fragrance.
6. Mix the liquid ingredients well. The oil and champagne will not stay mixed so mix just prior to step 7.
7. Add the liquid ingredients to your dry mixture of sodium bicarbonate and citric acid. When you add the liquid, you will see a little fizzing. This is because the sodium bicarbonate is reacting with the citric acid to produce carbon dioxide.
8. Using your hands, mix the liquid into the dry ingredients. When you have mixed the ingredients well there will be no dry areas and the colour will be even.
9. Begin to fill the flower moulds with the bath bomb mixture. Press the powder in firmly into each cavity to ensure the shape holds together.
10. After all the cavities have been filled, turn the bath bombs out onto some greaseproof paper.

*for a brighter coloured bath bomb, use cosmetic colour yellow (D&C Yellow No. 10- CI 47005). Substitute an equal amount of water for the food colouring and add the cosmetic pigment to the dry ingredients.

Elderflower & Ivy Honey Bath Bombs

Ingredients
800 g / 28 oz Sodium bicarbonate
400 g / 14 oz Citric acid
10 ml / 2 tsp Ivy honey
15 ml / 3 tsp Elderflower presse
10 ml / 2 tsp Ivy fragrance oil
10 ml / 2 tsp Sunflower oil
1 pinch Acid yellow 23 (CI 19140)
1 pinch Blue 1 lake (CI 42090)*

Equipment
A scoop
Weighing scales
Measuring spoons
Sieve
Large bowl
Small bowl
Leaf moulds
Gloves
Greaseproof paper

Making the Bath Bombs

1. Place your large bowl on the scales. Place the sieve on top of the bowl and zero the scale.
2. Wearing your gloves, scoop 800 g / 28 oz sodium bicarbonate into the sieve and sieve into the large bowl
3. Zero the scale again. Scoop 400 g / 14 oz of citric acid into the sieve. Sift the citric acid into the large bowl containing the sodium bicarbonate.
4. Add a pinch of the yellow and blue colour pigment to the bicarbonate and citric acid.
5. Mix the sodium bicarbonate, citric acid, yellow and blue pigment with your hands until the colour is mixed through evenly.
6. Into a small bowl measure the liquid ingredients: 15 ml / 3tsp elderflower presse, 10 ml / 2 tsp sunflower oil, 10 ml / 2 tsp ivy honey, and 10 ml / 2 tsp ivy fragrance
7. Mix the liquid ingredients well. The oil and elderflower presse will not stay mixed so mix just prior to step 8.
8. Add the liquid ingredients to your dry mixture of sodium bicarbonate and citric acid. When you add the liquid, you will see a little fizzing. This is because the sodium bicarbonate is reacting with the citric acid to produce carbon dioxide.
9. Using your hands, mix the liquid into the dry ingredients. When you have mixed the ingredients well there will be no dry areas and the couour will be even.
10. Begin to fill the leaf moulds with the bath bomb mixture. Press the powder in firmly into each cavity to ensure the shape holds together.
11. After all the cavities have been filled, turn the bath bombs out onto some greaseproof paper.

*if you do not have access to these cosmetic colours, you may substitute food colouring. Decrease the amount of water by the volume of food colouring added

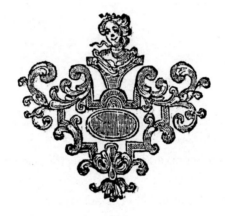

Chapter 6

Dr Sara's Beeswax Lip Balm

Handmade lip balm is easy to make and when made with unrefined beeswax is very healing for dry lips. Lip balm is made by mixing selected oils and wax together, melting the mixture and adding any desired flavour and colour. It is one of the easiest products to make. You can incorporate honey, however, this is difficult to do because honey is water soluble and does not easily mix with the oil base of the balm. When choosing colours and flavours, solubility is a major consideration. Use oil based flavours to add taste to your balms. Also, do not be tempted to try to add water based colours, they will not mix. Select oil dispersible pigments if you wish to add colour to handmade lip balms (see Table 1).

You need only a microwave or a bain-marie (double boiler), a Pyrex pitcher and a few lip balm pots and tubes to make lip balm. While it is not recommended to melt beeswax in a microwave, I find if the wax is added to the other lip balm ingredients, it melts well, without overheating. I put the oils and beeswax together for the base (omitting the colour and flavour) and put it into the microwave until all ingredients are liquid. This base can then be used to make a variety of flavoured lip balms of different colours. The colours recommended for lip balms include ultramarine pink and red iron oxide. To add sparkle to your lip balms, add mica powder

There are many oils which can be used to make lip balms. Very often commercial lip balms contain sweet almond oil. Almond oil is used because of its moisturizing properties. If however you are making lip balm for someone with a nut allergy, you would not want to include any nut oils in the recipe. I substitute sunflower oil and find the resulting product to be just as moisturizing.

The following recipes give a number of alternatives for lip balm base. They all are very easy to make however, you may find some of the ingredients are not easily to obtain available. I am sure you will find one you are pleased with. Any one of them can be used as a base to make flavoured lip balms.

Traditional Lip Balm Base

Ingredients	Equipment
110 g / 3.9oz Sweet almond oil	Weighing scales
50 g / 1.8 oz Cocoa butter	Bain-marie or microwave oven
20 g / 0.7 oz Unrefined beeswax	Small Pyrex measuring cup or glass bowl
	Plastic storage tub

Making the Lip balm base
1. Place your Pyrex measuring cup or glass bowl on the scale. Zero the scale to remove the weight of the container.
2. Place beeswax into the bowl until you have 20 g / 0.7 oz total weight.
3. Zero the scale again. Measure 50 g / 1.8 oz cocoa butter on the scale by adding the cocoa butter to the container.
4. Once again, zero the scale and weight 110 g / 3.9 oz sweet almond oil into the container.
5. Transfer the glass container to the top of the bain-marie or pan of water or put into the microwave.
6. Heat on medium heat until the beeswax and cocoa butter have melted completely
7. Stir the melted ingredients thoroughly with spoon.
8. Transfer the Lip balm base while still hot to the plastic storage container.

This recipe can be scaled up to meet your needs. Lip balm base can be melted in the microwave, colour and flavour added and then put into lip balm pots. This recipe used sweet almond oil as the liquid oil. While this is a very lovely Lip balm base remember this is not appropriate for those with nut allergies. The recipe which follows is a suitable substitution for this base and uses sunflower oil instead of sweet almond oil.

Sunflower Lip Balm Base

Ingredients
120 g / 4.2 oz Sunflower oil
40 g / 1.4 oz Cocoa butter
40 g / 1.4 oz Unrefined beeswax

Equipment
Weighing scales
Microwave oven or bain-marie
Small Pyrex measuring cup or glass bowl
Plastic storage tub

Making the Lip balm base
1. Place your Pyrex measuring cup or glass bowl on the scale. Zero the scale to remove the weight of the container.
2. Place beeswax into the bowl until you have 40 g / 1.4 oz total weight.
3. Zero the scale again. Measure 40 g / 1.4 oz cocoa butter on the scale by adding the cocoa butter to the container.
4. Once again, zero the scale and weight 120 g / 4.2 oz sunflower oil into the container.
5. Transfer the glass container to the bain-marie or microwave.
6. Heat on medium heat until the beeswax and cocoa butter have melted completely

7. Stir the melted ingredients thoroughly with spoon.
8. Transfer the Lip balm base while still hot to the plastic storage container.

Sunflower Lip balm base is a good substitution for the traditional Lip balm base. I use this most often as a base in my shop because it does not contain nut oil. This recipe can be scaled up to meet your needs. Lip balm base can be melted in the microwave, colour and flavour added and then put into lip balm pots.

Sunflower Base For Tubes

Ingredients
110 g / 3.9 oz Sunflower oil
45 g / 1.6 oz Cocoa butter
45 g / 1.6 oz Unrefined beeswax

Equipment
Weighing scales
Bain-marie or microwave
Small Pyrex measuring cup or glass bowl
Plastic storage tub

Making the Lip balm base
1. Place your Pyrex measuring cup or glass bowl on the scale. Zero the scale to remove the weight of the container.
2. Place beeswax into the bowl until you have 45 g / 1.6 oz total weight.
3. Zero the scale again. Measure 45 g / 1.6 oz cocoa butter on the scale by adding the cocoa butter to the container.
4. Once again, zero the scale and weight 110 g / 3.9 oz sunflower oil into the container.
5. Transfer the glass container to the top of the bain-marie or pan of water or put the bowl in the microwave.
6. Heat on medium heat until the beeswax and cocoa butter have melted completely
7. Stir the melted ingredients thoroughly with spoon.
8. Transfer the Lip balm base while still hot to the plastic storage container.

This base is ideal when making tubes of lip balm. It is slightly firmer and holds its form in the tube nicely. This recipe can be scaled up to meet your needs. Lip balm base can be melted in the microwave, colour and flavour added and then put into lip balm tubes.

Mango Butter Balm Base

Ingredients
110 g / 3.9 oz Sweet almond oil
20 g / 0.7 oz Mango butter
40 g / 1.4 oz Cocoa butter
30 g / 1.1 oz Unrefined beeswax

Equipment
Weighing scales
Microwave oven or bain-marie
Small Pyrex measuring cup or glass bowl
Plastic storage tub

Making the Lip balm base
1. Place your Pyrex measuring cup or glass bowl on the scale. Zero the scale to remove the weight of the container.
2. Place beeswax into the bowl until you have 30 g / 1.1 oz total weight.
3. Zero the scale again. Measure 40 g / 1.4 oz cocoa butter on the scale by adding the cocoa butter to the container.
4. Again, zero the scale again and measure 20 g / 0.7 oz mango butter on the scale by adding the cocoa butter to the container.
5. Once again, zero the scale and weight 110 g / 3.9 oz sweet almond oil into the container.
6. Transfer the glass container to the top of the bain-marie or microwave oven.
7. Heat on medium heat until the beeswax and cocoa butter have melted completely
8. Stir the melted ingredients thoroughly with spoon.
9. Transfer the Lip balm base while still hot to the plastic storage container.

I was very surprised the first time I saw mango butter. I think I expected an orange butter. It is a soft white butter made from the seed of the mango fruit. This recipe can be scaled up to meet your needs. Lip balm base can be melted in the microwave, colour and flavour added and then put into lip balm pots.

Shea Butter Balm Base

Ingredients
120 g / 4.2 oz Sweet almond oil
30 g / 1.1 oz Cocoa butter
20 g / 0.7 oz Shea butter
25 g / 0.9 oz Unrefined beeswax

Equipment
Weighing scales
Bain-marie
Small Pyrex measuring cup or glass bowl
Plastic storage tub

Making the Lip balm base
1. Place your Pyrex measuring cup or glass bowl on the scale. Zero the scale to remove the weight of the container.
2. Place beeswax into the bowl until you have 25 g / 0.9 oz total weight.
3. Zero the scale again. Measure 30 g / 1.1 oz cocoa butter on the scale by adding

the cocoa butter to the container.

4. After you zero the scale, measure 20 g / 0.7 oz of shea butter into the glass container.

5. Once again, zero the scale and weight 120 g / 4.2 oz sweet almond oil into the container.

6. Transfer the glass container to the top of the bain-marie or microwave oven.

7. Heat on medium heat until the beeswax, shea butter, and cocoa butter have melted completely.

8. Stir the melted ingredients thoroughly with spoon.

9. Transfer the Lip balm base while still hot to the plastic storage container.

Shea butter is also called African karite butter. While shea butter is very moisturizing, it can become grainy. This is not a result of the shae butter going off it is simply the shea butter fractionating. This lip balm may not be as smooth as the Mango Butter Base. This recipe can be scaled up to meet your needs. Lip balm base can be melted in the microwave, colour and flavour added and then put into lip balm pots.

Nutty Lip Balm Base

Ingredients	Equipment
60 g / 2.1 oz Sweet almond oil	Weighing scales
30 g / 1.1 oz Macadamia nut oil	Bain-marie or microwave oven
30 g / 1.1 oz Hazelnut oil	Small Pyrex measuring cup or glass
40 g / 1.4 oz Cocoa butter	bowl
40 g / 1.4 oz Unrefined beeswax	Plastic storage tub

Making the Lip balm base

1. Place your Pyrex measuring cup or glass bowl on the scale. Zero the scale to remove the weight of the container.

2. Place beeswax into the bowl until you have 40 g / 1.4 oz total weight.

3. Zero the scale again. Measure 40 g / 1.4 oz cocoa butter on the scale by adding the cocoa butter to the container.

4. Once again, zero the scale and weight 60 g / 2.1 oz sweet almond oil into the container.

5. Next, after the scale has been set back to zero, weigh 30 g / 1.1 oz hazelnut oil.

6. Weigh 30 g / 1.1 oz macadamia nut oil into the container after you have set the scale to zero.

7. Transfer the glass container to the top of the bain-marie or the microwave oven.

8. Heat on medium heat until the beeswax and cocoa butter have melted completely

9. Stir the melted ingredients thoroughly with spoon.
10. Transfer the Lip balm base while still hot to the plastic storage container.

This formulation has a wonderful nutty fragrance. You might want to put this directly into pots for use. Remember to label your Nutty Lip Balm as it is a big no-no for any one with a nut allergy. This recipe can be scaled up to meet your needs. Lip balm base can be melted in the microwave, colour and flavour added and then put into lip balm pots.

Coconut Lip Balm Base

Ingredients
80 g / 2.8 oz Sweet almond oil
30 g / 1.1 oz Cocoa butter
20 g / 0.7 oz Unrefined coconut oil
20 g / 0.7 oz Unrefined beeswax

Equipment
Weighing scales
Bain-marie or or the microwave oven
Small Pyrex measuring cup or glass bowl
Plastic storage tub

Making the Lip balm base
1. Place your Pyrex measuring cup or glass bowl on the scale. Zero the scale to remove the weight of the container.
2. Place beeswax into the bowl until you have 20 g / 0.7 oz total weight.
3. Zero the scale again. Measure 30 g / 1.1 oz cocoa butter on the scale by adding the cocoa butter to the container.
4. After you zero the scale, weigh 20 g / 0.7 oz unrefined coconut oil into the bowl.
5. finally, zero the scale and weigh 80 g / 2.8 oz sweet almond oil into the container.
6. Transfer the glass container to the top of the bain-marie or microwave oven.
7. Heat on medium heat until the beeswax and cocoa butter have melted completely
8. Stir the melted ingredients thoroughly with spoon.
9. Transfer the Lip balm base while still hot to the plastic storage container.

The smell of the unrefined coconut oil reminds me of cookies my mom used to make when I was a child. If you cannot get unrefined or virgin coconut oil, you can substitute refined coconut oil. Coconut lip balm is very nice as an unflavoured lip balm and can be put into pots immediately. Alternatively, coconut Lip balm base can be melted in the microwave, colour and flavour added and then put into lip balm pots. Remember, if you want more, this recipe can be scaled up to meet your needs.

Chapter 7

Making Flavoured Lip Balms

Unflavoured lip balms do the job they are intended to do, namely that they moisturize and protect your lips. Beeswax is the key to this healing process. Many of us enjoy having lip balm that is flavoured and coloured. Little girls love lip balms. I usually make a large pot of base lip balm and keep it handy then make smaller volumes of coloured and flavoured lip balms with the girls who come to my shop.

Adding colour to lip balm base is a little more difficult than adding flavour. The colours should be pigments and not water based colours. Water and oil do not mix. Table I suggests a number of colours which are suitable to use in lip balms. Remember pigment colours do not dissolve but disperse through the product. It is necessary to break the pigment into small particles in order to give a uniform appearance. To add the colour, melt the lip balm base and add a small amount of pigment colour. The amount of colour you should add will be a very small amount and below the amount you can weigh. Start with a small pinch. Stir to incorporate. Some of the colour may settle at the bottom. It is sometimes difficult to get all the pigment to disperse. You can either stir this in as the lip balm sets, or pour the balm into another container and leave this sediment in the first container. I tend to let the lip balm cool until it becomes like butter and continue to stir. I can usually get the pigment to break up and disperse through the balm. Then I re-melt the lip balm and if there is still sediment, I decant into another container. Add mica to your lip balm base using the same method. Again, only a tiny amount is needed to give a little sparkle. After I have incorporated the colour and have the desired shade, add the flavour.

To add flavour to lip balm base, all you need to do is melt the base and stir in the flavour. This is a very easy process. The only restriction is the flavour must be oil soluble. Water based flavours will not incorporate. Water based flavours are things like vanilla extract, lemon extract. These are usually in a solution containing alcohol and water, neither of which will mix with your lip balm base. I put the coloured base into the microwave just until the lip balm has melted and then add the desired flavour and stir. The lip balm is now ready to put into pots or tubes.

When pouring your lip balm into pots, start with very warm lip balm. I prefer to use a small Pyrex measuring jug because it has a lip which makes pouring easier. Pour into the pots and put aside to cool. Leave the lids off the pots until the lip balm has cooled completely. You should get a very smooth top which looks very professional. To pour into tubes, pour lip balm to fill the tube approximately three quarters of the way to the top. Set this aside and let the balm cool completely. Give the lip balm a twist in the tube to loosen it from the turning mechanism. Turn back to the lowest position. You will need to re-melt the lip balm. Only heat until it has melted enough to pour into the tubes. Fill the tube to the top with melted lip balm. By pouring the lip balm in two stages, you will have a flat appearance when the second volume has cooled. This little trick will give you perfect tubes if done with care.

You are limited only by your imagination when it comes to combining lip balm base, colour and flavour. Following are a few suggested combinations.

Sugar Plum Kiss

Ingredients:
50 g / 1.8 oz Lip balm base
1 pinch of Ultramarine pink
2.5 ml/ ½ tsp Raspberry flavour oil

Equipment:
Microwave oven or bain-marie
Small Pyrex measuring cup
Spoon
½ tsp Measuring spoon
10- 5 ml Lip balm pots

Making the Lip Balm
1. Place the Pyrex jug on the scale and zero the scale. Weigh 50 g / 1.8oz lip balm base into a Pyrex measuring jug with a pouring spout.
2. Melt the base in the microwave or bain-marie.
3. Add a pinch of ultramarine pink to the base. Stir to incorporate.
4. Add 2.5 ml or ½ tsp raspberry flavour to the melted base and stir.
5. Pour Sugar Plum Kiss into the lip balm pots while the lip balm is melted.

Coconut lip balm base, sunflower lip balm base or mango butter base work well.

Pink Lemonade Kiss

Ingredients:
100 g / 3.6 oz Lip balm base
1 pinch of Manganese violet
2.5 ml/ ½ tsp Lemon flavour oil
2.5ml/ ½ tsp Srawberry flavour oil
1 pinch of Mica

Equipment:
Microwave or on bain-marie.
Small Pyrex measuring cup
Spoon
½ tsp Measuring spoon
20- 5 ml Lip balm pots

Making the Lip Balm

1. Place the Pyrex jug on the scale and zero the scale. Weigh 100 g / 3.6 oz Lip balm base into a Pyrex measuring jug with a pouring spout.
2. Melt the base in the microwave or on bain-marie.
3. Add a pinch of magnesium violet and a pinch of mica to the base. Stir to incorporate. You may need to mix until balm cools slightly and re-melt.
4. Add 2.5 ml or ½ tsp lemon flavour and 2.5 ml or ½ tsp strawberry flavour to the melted base and stir.
5. Pour the Pink Lemonade Kiss into the lip balm pots while the lip balm is melted.

Sunflower lip balm base, traditional lip balm base or mango butter base work well.

Orange Blossom Balm

Ingredients:
100 g / 3.6 oz Lip balm base
2.5 ml/ ½ tsp Orange flavour oil
2.5ml/ ½ tsp Carrot oil
1 pinch Mica

Equipment:
Microwave or bain-marie
Small Pyrex measuring cup
Spoon
½ tsp Measuring spoon
10- 5 ml Lip balm pots

Making the Lip Balm

1. Place the Pyrex jug on the scale and zero the scale. Weigh 100 g / 3.6 oz lip balm base into a Pyrex measuring jug with a pouring spout.
2. Melt the base in the microwave or on bain-marie.
3. Add 2.5 ml or ½ tsp orange flavour and 2.5 ml or ½ tsp carrot oil to the melted base and stir.
4. Pour orange blossom balm into the lip balm pots while the lip balm is melted.

Shea butter base, sunflower lip balm base or traditional lip balm base work well.

Peppermint Kiss

Ingredients:
50 g / 1.8 oz Lip balm base
1 pinch of Ultramarine blue
1 pinch Mica
2.5 ml/ ½ tsp peppermint Flavour oil

Equipment:
Microwave or bain-marie
Small Pyrex measuring cup
Spoon
½ tsp Measuring spoon
20- 5 ml Lip balm pots

Making the Lip Balm

1. Place the Pyrex jug on the scale and zero the scale. Weigh 50 g / 1.8 oz lip balm base into a Pyrex measuring jug with a pouring spout.
2. Melt the base in the microwave or on bain-marie.
3. Add a pinch of ultramarine blue and a pinch of mica to the base. Stir to incorporate. You may need to mix until balm cools slightly and re-melt.
4. Add 2.5 ml or ½ tsp peppermint flavour to the melted base and stir.
5. Pour the Peppermint Kiss into the lip balm pots while the lip balm is melted.

Sunflower lip balm base, shea butter base or mango butter base work well.

Vanilla Bean Balm

Ingredients:
50 g / 1.8 oz Lip balm base
2.5 ml/ ½ tsp Vanilla flavour oil

Equipment:
Microwave or bain-marie
Small Pyrex measuring cup
Spoon
½ tsp Measuring spoon
10- 5 ml Lip balm pots

Making the Lip Balm

1. Place the Pyrex jug on the scale and zero the scale. Weigh 50 g / 1.8oz lip balm base into a Pyrex measuring jug with a pouring spout.
2. Melt the base in the microwave or on bain-marie.
3. Add 2.5 ml or ½ tsp vanilla flavour to the melted base and stir.
4. Pour Vanilla Bean into the lip balm pots while the lip balm is melted.

Coconut lip balm base, sunflower lip balm base or nutty lip base work well.

White Chocolate Cherry Lip Balm

Ingredients:
100 g / 3.6 oz Lip balm base
1 Pinch of Manganese Violet
2.5 ml/ ½ tsp Cherry flavour oil
2.5ml/ ½ tsp Vanilla flavour oil

Equipment:
Microwave or bain-marie
Small Pyrex measuring cup
Spoon
½ tsp Measuring spoon
20- 5 ml Lip balm pots

Making the Lip Balm

1. Place the Pyrex jug on the scale and zero the scale. Weigh 100 g / 3.6 oz lip balm base into a Pyrex measuring jug with a pouring spout.

2. Melt the base in the microwave or on bain-marie.
3. Add a pinch of magnesium violet and a pinch of mica to the base. Stir to incorporate. You may need to mix until balm cools slightly and re-melt.
4. Add 2.5 ml or ½ tsp cherry flavour and 2.5 ml or ½ tsp vanilla flavour to the melted base and stir.
5. Pour the White Chocolate Cherry Lip Balm into the lip balm pots while the lip balm is melted.

Nutty lip balm base, traditional lip balm base or mango butter base work well.

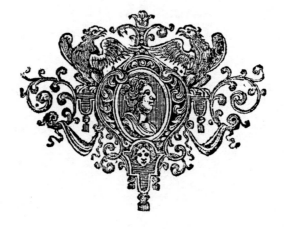

Chapter 8

Introduction To Traditional Soap Making

Soapmaking is a very old craft. People have been making soap using various methods through the centuries. The two ingredients necessary to make soap are fatty acids and hydroxide. In the past soap would have been made with animal fats (the fatty acids), such as tallow or lard and a crudely isolated form of hydroxide, or potassium hydroxide. The soapmaker would have collected ashes from the fire and leached the hydroxide from them by running water through the ashes. Next, the soapmaker would try to determine if the lye was of the correct concentration. The methods of assessing lye concentration included putting an egg or potato into the solution to see if either would float. If the egg or potato was suspended just below halfway the solution was the correct concentration to make soap. Instead of an egg or potato, sometimes a feather was used. If a chicken feather dissolved in the lye, then the solution was ready to make soap. If these tests revealed the lye solution was not strong enough, then the liquid was reduced until it passed the potato or feather test. Once the lye solution was ready, the soapmaking could begin. The fat would have been mixed with the lye to make the soap. This mixture may have been stirred over heat to get the soap to form. After the soap mixture had thickened some, it would have been poured into moulds and left to sit. Eventually it would have been taken out of the moulds, the soap would have been cut into pieces and then left to cure until the water content of the soap had reduced. Results probably varied. The problem with this method was the early soapmaker really did not know what the concentration of hydroxide was in the solution. As a result, it would have been very difficult to get the proportions correct to make a good soap. Too little hydroxide, and the soap was a soft, greasy mass, too much hydroxide, and the soap was caustic and could burn skin. To test if the soap was safe to use and non-caustic, soapmakers used to touch the soap to their tongue. If the soap burned their tongue, the soap was caustic and should not be used. If the soap did not burn the soapmakers tongue, then the soap was safe to use and the cleaning could begin.

Thankfully, soapmaking has moved on from these days. The soapmaker no longer must leach ashes for lye or use such inaccurate methods for testing the concentration of the lye solution. The manufacture of chemicals has given soapmakers sodium hydroxide, a form of hydroxide which produces a harder bar of soap than that produced by potassium hydroxide. Sodium hydroxide has replaced potassium hydroxide in the manufacture of bars of soap, while potassium hydroxide continues to be used in liquid soap production. Finally, we are no longer restricted to the fats from the animals on the farm. Today there is a wide selection of oils in the grocery stores, many of which are exotic. Soapmaking has become a craft which can be widely pursued.

Soap is still made by treating oils and fats with a strong alkali in the form of an aqueous hydroxide solution, commonly called lye. Let us consider the ingredients used to make soap:

Water

The water that you use will influence the quality of the finished soap. Very often soap recipes call for deionised water or some other pure form such as rainwater. I love the idea of making soap with rainwater however this may not always be possible. Additionally, many recipes say that tap water may never be used. If you have hard water, you probably should avoid using tap water because of the high calcium content. If your water is soft, then you can very likely make a good soap with your tap water. When I began making soap, I thought about consistency when I selected my water source. As I was pretty sure I would not live in my flat for the rest of my soap making days, I decided that I would not use my tap water. I imagined making very nice soap for a number of years with my tap water and then moving home and making a seemingly trivial change to the new tap water only to discover the soap does not work the way it used to. I recommend that whatever source of water you use, be consistent or at least realize that by changing your source of water, you may change the quality of the soap. Recipes also steer the soapmaker away from any water that contains minerals and ions. I make my soap with mineral water and am very pleased with the result. I have tried a number of different mineral waters and recommend avoiding those with high calcium.

Sodium Hydroxide/Lye/Hydroxide

Sodium hydroxide is the chemical indicated by the notation $NaOH$ and commonly called caustic soda. You may have this in your house. It is often used to unblock drains. If you do not have sodium hydroxide, you can purchase this at your local chemists, or at a hardware store. While sodium hydroxide is a common household chemical, it is a chemical and safety should be observed. Please read the safety warning on the label. Lye refers to hydroxide dissolved in water. The lye is the potion that converts the oil to soap. Sodium hydroxide reacts with the oil to make glycerine and soap. Lye is a strong alkali solution. When making solid soap bars, the lye solution is made with sodium hydroxide. When making liquid soap, it is most often potassium hydroxide that is used the lye solution. It is the hydroxide that reacts with the oils and fats in the chemical reaction of saponification to produce soap. The sodium and potassium do not participate in the chemical reaction, but combine with the soap molecules as salts. It is important to understand it is the hydroxide that is reacting with the oil.

When you purchase sodium hydroxide for soapmaking, check the purity. Look for sodium hydroxide that is 98%. Some cheaper sodium hydroxide products sold in discount shops may be adequate for opening a drain, but will not be appropriate for making soap. I have had students who have purchased sodium hydroxide which did not indicate the purity on the container. This sodium hydroxide did not work in the soap formulations. I suspect it is because it is a much lower percent of sodium hydroxide

Oils and fats

Soap can be made from plant oils, such as olive and coconut oils, as well as animal fats, such as lard and tallow. Plant oils and animal fats are chemically similar. Both are composed of mixtures of different triglycerides. A triglyceride is simply a glycerine molecule with three fatty acids covalently connected to it.

$$CH_2-O-\overset{\overset{\displaystyle O}{\|}}{C}-(CH_2)_{14}-CH_3$$

$$CH-O-\overset{\overset{\displaystyle O}{\|}}{C}-(CH_2)_{14}-CH_3$$

$$CH_2-O-\overset{\overset{\displaystyle O}{\|}}{C}-(CH_2)_{14}-CH_3$$

Triglyceride

In each triglyceride molecule, the three fatty acid molecules can be different and these differences depend upon the oil source. So the triglycerides in olive oil are different from the triglycerides in coconut oil. Additionally the triglyceride composition of any given oil will vary from crop to crop. So olive oil produced one year will vary slightly from olive oil produced in another year. Also olive oil grown in one location will have a slightly different triglyceride composition than that grown in another area. This composition is important in the formulation of soap recipes.

The Chemistry of Soapmaking

The chemical reaction of saponification is the reaction of triglycerides with hydroxide to yield soap and glycerine. The hydroxide molecule reacts to release the fatty acid from the glycerine back bone. One hydroxide is needed to "cut" each of the three fatty acid side chains. To react one triglyceride molecule, you need three molecules of hydroxide because there are three fatty acids in each triglyceride. The hydroxide is incorporated into the products and the result is synthesis of one glycerine molecule and three molecules of soap in the form of a sodium salt. Below is an example in which a palm oil triglyceride is reacted with three molecules of sodium hydroxide to produce a glycerol molecule, also called glycerine, and three molecules of palm oil soap, or sodium palmitate.

Triglyceride   Glycerol

In order to formulate a soap recipe, we need to calculate how much sodium hydroxide we need to react with the oils we are using. The sodium hydroxide has a constant weight, while the triglyceride molecule's weight depends upon which fatty acids make up the side chains. As mentioned earlier, not only does the triglyceride composition vary by oil but also from crop to crop. Because of this, the amount of sodium hydroxide needed in the saponification reaction is determined empirically for each specific oil. This amount is then expressed as a saponification value.

The Saponification Value

The saponification value, also called a SAP value, is expressed as the milligrams of potassium hydroxide (KOH) required to saponify 1 gram of a specific oil. The SAP value differs for each plant oil and animal fat and must be determined empirically. This is done by experimentally reacting the oil with potassium hydroxide to determine the number of milligrams required to convert one gram of that oil to soap. Appendix 1 lists the SAP Values in the correct units of mg hydroxide / gram oil for a number of oils used to make soap. Most soapmakers do not work in milligrams when making soap so it makes since to convert the amount of hydroxide needed into grams. To do this, we divide by 1000 because there are 1000 mg in each gram. This calculation gives us a factor we can use to formulate our recipe in grams.

200 mg KOH / g Palm Oil ÷ 1000 mg/g = 0.200 g KOH/g Palm Oil
0.200 g KOH/g Palm Oil = the KOH Factor

For instance, the potassium hydroxide SAP value for palm oil is 200 mg KOH to saponifly 1 g palm oil. In this case, the SAP value of 200 mg KOH/ gram palm oil has been divided by 1000 to convert to 0.200 grams KOH to per gram palm oil. We can call the grams needed to convert one gram of palm oil the KOH Factor. This is listed in appendix I one as well. As mentioned above, when we make solid soap, we use sodium hydroxide rather than potassium hydroxide. We calculate a NAOH Factor to use when formulating recipes with sodium hydroxide. To convert the KOH Factor to the NaOH Factor, the KOH Factor is divided by the ratio of the molecular weights of potassium hydroxide. The molecular weight of KOH is 56.11 g/mol and the molecular weight of sodium hydroxide, NaOH is 40.0 g/mol.

To calculate the ratio:
56.11g/mol ÷ 40.0 g/mol = 1.403 conversion factor

To convert to the NaOH SAP value for palm oil, we do the following:

0.200 KOH Factor ÷ 1.403 conversion factor = 0.143 NaOH Factor

The NaOH Factor is used to correctly formulate soap recipes using sodium hydroxide as our alkili. If, for instance we want to saponify 100 g of palm oil using sodium hydroxide, the NaOH Factor allows us to calculate how much sodium hydroxide we need to convert the total amount of oil into soap. In practice, we do not want to convert all the oil or fat into soap but would like to leave a percentage of the oils or fats in their natural form. This is called superfatting.

Superfatting

Soap which is superfatted is soap which is made by a recipe which results in some of the oils remaining as oils, rather than being saponified into soap and glycerin. Soap is frequently superfatted by 5%, 9%, 15% and so on. The percentage refers to the percentage of oils which are not converted into soap. The two main methods of superfatting a soap recipe is to add excess oil to the soap recipe after adding the amount of hydroxide needed to saponify the total oils in your recipe. The other method is to calculate the amount of lye needed to completely saponify all the oil and then decrease or discount the sodium hydroxide by a percentage. Superfatting adds moisture to the soap by leaving some of the oil. An added benefit of superfatting is it gives you a safety margin when making your soap. As mentioned, we do not want excess hydroxide in the finished soap because it can burn the skin.

Let us consider three examples.

Example 1

> We have 100 g palm oil with a NaOH Factor of 0.143 g NaOH/ gram of palm oil.
> 100 g palm oil × 0.143 g NaOH/gram palm oil = 14.3 g NaOH

This calculation shows us that we need 14.3 grams NaOH to convert all of the 100 grams of palm oil to soap and glycerine. Figure 1 represents a situation where we add the exact amount of NaOH needed to change all the palm oil into soap.

Figure 1

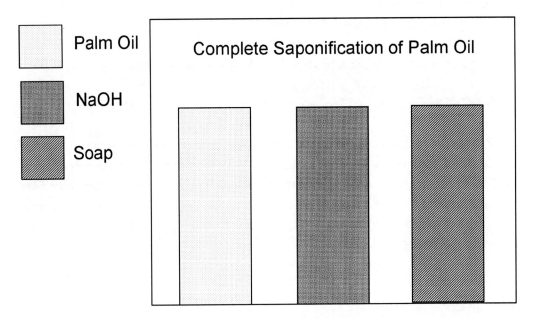

In Figure 1 we see that there is the exact amount of sodium hydroxide as is needed to convert all the palm oil to soap. As a result, there is no remaining palm oil and all the NaOH is consumed. This represents a theoretical situation. Soapmakers never make soap that is 0% superfatted. This is a simplified representation not taking into account the three to one ratio of hydroxide needed in the chemical reaction

Example 2

> Once again, we have 100 g palm oil with a NaOH Factor of 0.143 g NaOH/ gram of palm oil. However, in this example, we would like the soap to be 10 % superfatted.

> 100 g palm oil × 0.143 g NaOH/gram palm oil = 14.3 g NaOH

Next we multiply the amount of NaOH by 0.9 to calculate how much NaOH we need to have 90% of the total.

14.3 grams NaOH x 0.9 = 12.9 grams NaOH

These calculations show us that we need 12.9 grams NaOH to convert 90% of the 100 g of palm oil to soap and glycerine.

Figure 2

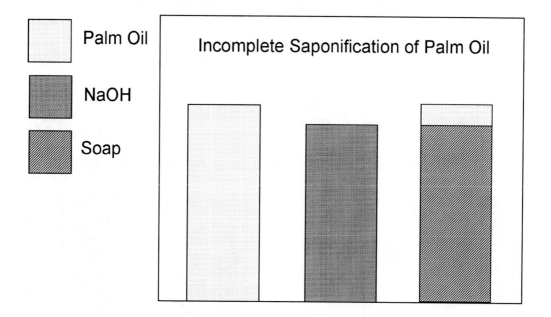

Figure 2 represents a situation where we add the amount of NaOH needed to convert 90% the palm oil into soap and leave 10% in oil form. In this case, there is no residual sodium hydroxide, however, the soap is supperfatted by 10%, or 10 grams of the 100 grams of palm oil are unsaponificated. You can see on the far right there are both palm oil and soap visually represented in the chart. This is a simplified representation not taking into account the three to one ratio of hydroxide needed in the chemical reaction

Example 3

This example is intended to show you what can happen if you get the calulation incorrect or make a mistake measuring. Imagine you use the KOH Factor in your calculation and use NaOH in your recipe. We have 100 g palm oil with an NaOH Factor of 0.143 g NaOH/ gram of palm oil, however, we mistakenly use the KOH Factor of 0.200 g / gram of palm oil.

100 g palm oil × 0.200 g KOH /gram palm oil = 20.0 g KOH

Remember, 20 grams is the amount we would need to completely convert 100grams of palm oil to soap if we were using potassium hydroxide. While, 14.3 grams is the amount we we would need if we were using sodium hydroxide.

Let's say we continue with 20g and decide to supperfat by 10%
20.0 grams × 0.9 = 2.0 grams
20.0 g-2.0g=18.0 grams

In this example, we make the soap with 100 grams of palm oil and 18.0 grans NaOH. The mistake is we calculated with the KOH Factor. Figure 3 shows graphically what happens.

Figure 3

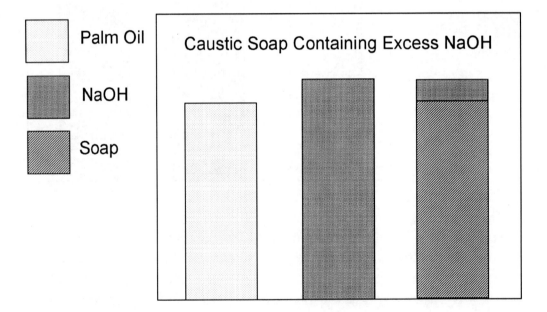

Because we used the incorrect factor in our formulation we make caustic soap. Even if we superfat by 10% in this example and decrease the amount from 20 g to 18 grams, because we calculated to use KOH and used NaOH, we will have an excess of hydroxide. All the palm oil is converted to soap, the extra hydroxide remains and there is no unreacted oil. This will result in a caustic product as depicted in figure 3. This soap will burn your skin, if used.

When making our soap, we would like to make soap as described in Example 2. We would like to have some of our oils unreacted so the soap is superfatted, safe to use and the resulting soap moisturizing. Appendix I lists the correct factors for making soap with both potassium hydroxide, the KOH Factor and with sodium hydroxide, the NaOH Factor. Appendix II is a soapmaking worksheet you can use to formulate your own soap. The soapmaking worksheet also lets you calculate the amount of hydroxide to use in order to superfat at 6%, 10% and 15%. Next I will describe my soapmaking method.

Chapter 9

Dr Sara's Easy Soapmaking Method

My interest in soapmaking began when I was a child in Iowa. My parents had a series of craft books in their library. I remember on cold winter days looking through the craft series hoping to find something to do on a cold Iowan snow day. Repeatedly, I would look through the book which described candle making and soap making. I was intrigued by the idea of making soaps. I still remember the descriptions of how to make the soap. The recipe called for coconut oil, something I could not even imagine. These were the days before the internet and so there was not an opportunity to go online and order the ingredients in the recipe. I was also impressed by the equipment needed to make soap, including thermometers, special pots and jars, all of which were things I did not have access to. Even so, I spent hours pouring over the soapmaking method with great curiosity. This intrigue about soapmaking did not disappear. When I was working on my PhD at Hershey Medical School, I bought a soapmaking book. Once again, I spent hours with the book, studying the method, the ingredients and the recipes. Even though I spent at least eight hours a day in a laboratory, often doing very complicated experiments, I did not feel I could make soap. The description made it sound very dangerous. Additionally, there was a requirement for specialist equipment. As a graduate student, I did not have the extra money to invest in thermometers and pots, or to order the oils necessary to make soap so my interest in soapmaking was again set aside.

Time passed, I completed my degree, and moved on to my post-doctorate position in Scotland. Because my post-doctorate fellowship was a short term position, I only moved the bare minimum to the United Kingdom. The soapmaking book was left behind in America. As so often happens, my plans changed. After being in the UK for a few years, I got married. Shortly thereafter, our daughter Jasmine was born. Having Jasmine changed my life. I no longer desired to continue with my career in science. I was on the lookout for an alternative career, one I could do in my home with my beautiful daughter by my side. At the time, I considered making cookies. Starting a cookie company would have been easy in that I knew how to bake a number of delicious cookies that people would enjoy. The difficulty was that I had a new baby. Baking to order was not going to work. Believe it or not babies do not always cooperate in such ventures! I do not really know how soap came to mind but I decided my maternity leave would be a wonderful opportunity to finally learn to make soap. After all, soap is non-perishable and can be made at your convenience and stored. Convinced this was the way forward and would lead to my working at home with Jasmine by my side, I bought a second copy to the soapmaking book I had in America.

Once I had the soapmaking book, I needed to get the ingredients and the equipment. I bought 2 thermometers, ordered some palm oil and found the other oils at the local shops. I was able to get sodium hydroxide at my local chemist. I was ready to make soap. The kitchen became the soap laboratory. Jasmine would sit in her bouncy chair and I would make soap. It became habit for me to tell her all the steps in the process. Initially, I followed all the instructions meticulously. Even so, the results were not that consistent. I measured the temperature of both the oils and the lye very carefully. I stirred the exact amount of time and watched for the reaction to occur. I poured the soap mixture into the mould at the time the recipe told me to. With some practice, I finally was getting something which resembled soap.

However, I did not feel the method was leading to the results described. I was beginning to get a bit fed up with the methodology. I wondered how much of the method was required. As a scientist, I knew that some parts were probably not as important as others, so I began to experiment. Soapmaking as a craft is constantly evolving. Previously I mentioned an early method of soapmaking with ashes and animal fats. Now we can use a variety of oils and have access to very pure forms of hydroxide. If you investigate the methods available to make soap you will find a variety of techniques including hot-processed soap, cold processed soap, and others. When I began to make soap, I decided to use the cold-processed soapmaking method. This method does not add any external heat to the soap as it is being made. Cold processed soap methods require the use of thermometers in the process. Both the oil mixture and the lye are brought to the same temperature prior to being mixed together. I found this very tedious and began to think about soapmaking through history. I doubt early soapmakers had access to thermometers and so I thought you must be able to make soap without measuring the temperatures of the lye and oils.

The first thing I did was get rid of the thermometers and quit stirring the length of time the recipe suggested. I stirred with my stick mixer until the soap mixture became thick. To my surprise, the soap recipes still worked. I actually began to get more consistent results from recipe to recipe. Next, I began to experiment with the lye concentrations. I had read that you can decrease the amount of water used in the lye solution. I increased the lye concentration until I was using a 36 % w/w solution. It is important to mention that I did not increase the amount of hydroxide, but decreased the amount of water the hydroxide was dissolved into. I found I was getting very good soap that processed very quickly. The maximum solubility of sodium hydroxide in water is around 52 % w/w so I was very far away from a saturated solution. However I stopped at 36 % w/w. In fact, the soap was processing so quickly it was hard and at a safe pH after it cooled.

As I experimented, I developed a method by which you can make soap without measuring the temperature of the oils or the lye. Using a lye solution that is 36%w/w it takes only a few minutes to get the soap to thicken or to trace and after it is poured into the mould, the soap processes incredibly rapidly. Finally, the resulting soap is firm and at a safe pH within hours of being taken from the pan. The soapmaking method presented in this book is a result of Jasmine and my soapmaking experiments.

Equipment

The equipment you need to make soap with my method, is equipment you may likely have or at least are items that are easily obtainable without great expense. You will need a scale. I recommend a digital scale that measures in increments of 1 gram. The more accurate the scale you use to weigh your ingredients, the greater consistency you will have in your soaps. It is vital that an accurate scale is used to weigh the water, sodium hydroxide, and oils used in the soap recipe. These simply cannot be accurately be measured by volume.

Once you have weighed the oils, you will need a way to melt those which are solid at room temperature. Today the easiest way to do this is to use a microwave oven. If you do not have a microwave oven, then the oils can be melted in a double boiler or bain-marie. Melting the solid oils eases the mixing of these oils with the liquid oils in preparation for mixing the lye solution with the oils.

Finally, you will benefit tremendously by having a stick mixer or electric hand mixer. In theory, you can make soap by stirring by hand. However, it will take a very long time to stir and is simply not worth the trouble. The hand blender has the advantage of mixing very quickly. When the oils and the lye are mixed together with a hand mixer, the molecules come into contact more quickly and the chemical reaction of saponification gets going more quickly. As saponification occurs, the reaction produces heat and this too makes the molecules intereact more quickly resulting in a mixture that thickens easily and is at a good temperature when it is poured into the pan. This heat will stay within the pan and process the soap in a speedy manor.

You will also need glass bowls, a heavy jar or Pyrex measuring cup and wooden spoon to prepare the lye, cling film, rubber gloves and some towels. Most of these items you will have in your kitchen. Again, you may wish to dedicate some of these items solely for soapmaking. For instance, the wooden spoon will get a bit beat up after a few uses to mix the lye. Also, if you are going to use anything plastic, it may retain the fragrance you put in the soap and so would not be suitable for food.

Dr Sara's Soapmaking Methodology:

The first thing I do is make the lye solution. I begin by weighing the water into a heavy glass jar with an accurate scale. I next weigh the sodium hydroxide or NaOH. I pour the NaOH into the water and stir until the hydroxide is completely dissolved. I them put the lye solution to the side and get the oils ready. I do not worry about the temperature of the hydroxide solution. In fact I sometimes make the lye a day before and use it cold to make the soap. I find it still works.

The next step is to get the oils ready. I measure all the oils I am going to use by weight. If the oil is a solid, such as coconut or palm, I weight these into a glass bowl and then transfer this to the microwave. I heat the solid oils only to the point where they are liquid. I am not trying to reach a certain temperature when I heat the oil, I am simply trying to melt the solid oils so I can mix them easily with the liquid oils and with the lye solution. After all the oils have been weighed and melted, I put them into a large glass bowl and stir them together. The oils are now ready to go.

It is time to begin adding the lye solution to the oil mixture. I slowly pour the lye solution into the bowl containing the oil mixture while stirring with a stick blender with the power off. After I have added all the llye solution, I begin to mix with the power on. I continue to stir until the soap mixture begins to thicken. It thickens quickly. It will begin at a consistency like a thin sauce, continue to thicken until it is like custard and will then resemble a thick batter. When it reaches the thickness of batter, it is time to stir in the additional ingredients. I add my fragrance and continue to stir.

I stir until the soap mixture is thick enough that a bit drizzled across the top creates a line. The soap is said to be at "trace" when you can see this line. The oils are well on their way to being converted to soap. I pour the soap into a mould. Most often I use a 9x9 baking pan that has been greased with palm oil. I cover the pan with cling film and then cover this with a number of towels to keep the heat in. The soap will continue to heat up and thicken. This is the chemical reaction occurring. It really is like putting a cake in the oven but you do not need to add heat. The soap will continue to warm until it heats up from the centre to the edges resembling a gel. This heat and gelling is a result of the chemical processing of the oils into soap by the lye. This may take an hour to complete.

You will be able to see the progression of the gel from the centre to the edges of the soap as it heats up. This is the saponification reaction converting the oil to soap from the centre to the edge of the pan. Once the reaction and the gel has reached the edge of the pan, I unwrap the soap and allow it to cool.

Once cool, the soap should be very solid. I sometimes put the soap in the freezer for a while to cool it more quickly. When it is cool, you should be able to turn the soap out of the container. I cut the soap into pieces and check the pH. The pH is usually around 9.

The next chapter has a number of basic soap recipes using this method. My soapmaking has been described as magic. The effort is in the preparation. It takes longer to weigh the ingredients than to actually mix the soap.

If I am going to make soap in small moulds, I sometimes increase the amount of water and decrease the lye concentration. The Soapmaking Worksheet in Appendix 2 shows how to formulate lye solutions at 30% w/w, 33% w/w, and 36% w/w.

Chapter 10

Basic Soap Recipes

In the last chapter I described my soapmaking methodology. Now it is time to make soap. The following recipes are simple recipes without any colour or fragrance. These basic soap recipes will give you an idea of which parts of the recipe are fixed and which parts are flexible. As mentioned earlier, each oil has its own saponification value and so cannot be substituted without risk of resulting in an inappropriate amount of sodium hydroxide (see examples 1 and 2). You can make unscented soap with these recipes, or you can add colour and fragrance. Unscented soaps, without additions, are ideal for people with fragrance sensitivities. The addition of colour and fragrance does not influence this formulation. So any basic soap recipe can be used to make endless varieties of soaps. I have often heard people say, I cannot make this recipe because I do not have that essential oil or fragrance. The fragrance does not influence the soap formulation and so any fragrance can be substituted.

I too was unsure about what ingredients were fixed in a soap making recipe. I remember looking through the recipe book and not having all the ingredients listed so not making a particular recipe. I now realize there are 2 parts to each soap recipe. The first part is the basic soap and the second part consists of the additional ingredients. The basic soap is made of the oils and sodium hydroxide. These ingredients participate in the saponification chemistry, and are fixed. The additional ingredients, while they may add qualities to the soap such as colour, fragrance and texture, they do not influence the chemistry, and are flexible. Because they are not involved in the saponification, they can be omitted or substituted with other ingredients. Once you realize this you will look at each recipe in a new way. You will identify the two parts of the recipe.

You can create a variety of luxurious soaps by adding various combinations of fragrance, spice, botanicals and colours to any basic soap recipe. When you are deciding on which additional ingredients to use in your soap, think about what you want the final soap to look like, feel like and smell like. Table 4 gives you some ideas of thinks you can add to the soap base recipes.

The addition of fragrance will give your soap a nice aroma. Other additions, which may add fragrance, are spices and teas. Spices can create a number of interesting colours as well as aroma. Herbal teas can add subtle fragrance, texture and colour to soaps. The addition of honey will give soap a light, sugary smell, make soap very moisturising and turn the soap a golden colour. You can add more than one of the listed additions to the soap base. Be creative and have fun choosing.

Suggested Combinations

Lavender Chamomile Soap
Additional ingredients: lavender essential oil, chamomile tea, ultramarine purple

Summer Garden Soap;
Additional ingredients: rose and raspberry tea, rose fragrance

Honey Spice Soap
Additional Ingredients: crystallized honey, cinnamon, nutmeg, fragrance

Table 4

Additives to add to Base Soap Recipes		
Additive	**Amount**	**Quality**
Essential Oil	15 ml/ 1 T	Fragrance
Fragrance Oil	30 ml/ 2 T	Fragrance
Honey	15 ml/ 1 T	Emollient
Colourant	See Chapter 2	Colour
Spice Powder[a]	5ml/ 1 tsp	Colour & Fragrance
Herbal Tea[b]	1- 2 sachets	Colour, Fragrance & texture
Rolled Oats	45 ml/ 3 T	Texture
Grated Beeswax	10 grams / 0.4oz	Emollient
Grains, Seeds, Rice Powder[c]	15 ml/ 1 T	Exfoliating

a   Spice powder can be used to add colour, texture and fragrance to soap. Recommended spices include; cinnamon, ginger, nutmeg, turmeric, or paprika.

b   Tea is a wonderful botanical addition to soap. It is recommended you use herbal and fruit teas rather than the darker teas like Earl Grey. For instance, chamomile, elderflower, blackberry, raspberry, dandelion, and even thistle tea works very well in soap.

c   The addition of seeds, grains or rice powder can add texture to soap to create an exfoliating bar. You can mix these all the way through the soap or just sprinkle the top of the soap to create soap with a moisturising side and an exfoliating side. A good source for rice powder is baby rice.

Basic Recipe 1 - Olive, Sunflower, Palm & Coconut

This is the basic soap recipe I use most often. It is a bit unconventional as it is very high in coconut oil and also is highly superfatted. I have read that too much coconut oil can be drying but with the high percentage of unsaponified oils this soap is extremely moisturizing and super bubbly. This is definitely my favourite basic recipe. Before you begin, gather the equipment and ingredients you will need. Also prepare your soap pan. If it is a plastic container, the soap will come out nicely. If you are using a metal pan, you may wish to grease the pan with a little palm oil to keep the soap from sticking.

Equipment	*Ingredients*
Scales	112 g or 4 oz Sodium hydroxide
Rubber gloves	(NaOH)
Large glass jar or a Pyrex measuring cup	200 g / 7 oz Water
Small plastic or glass bowl	150 g / 5.3 oz Olive oil
Large glass bowl	125 g / 4.4 oz Sunflower oil
Pan (9x9 inch)	175 g / 6.2 oz Palm oil
Wooden spoon	468 g / 16.5 oz Coconut oil
Electric stick mixer	
Microwave oven or bain-Marie	
Cling film	
Towels	
Spatula	

Making the Lye Solution

Lye Solution	
Water	**Sodium Hydroxide (NaOH)**
200 grams / 7 oz	112 grams / 4 oz
Safety Advice: Always add sodium hydroxide to water!	

1. Put on your rubber gloves before you begin.
2. Place the large glass jar or Pyrex measuring cup on the scale and tare (re-zero) the scale to eliminate the jar weight.
3. Weigh the water into the jar so the water weight is 200 g or 7 oz.
4. Put the jar of water to the side.
5. Place the small plastic or glass bowl on the scale and re-zero the scale. Carefully pour the sodium hydroxide into the bowl until you have 112 g or 4oz of sodium hydroxide.

6. Move to sink and place water jar in the sink. Slowly pour the sodium hydroxide into the large jar containing the water. You can swirl the jar to begin mixing the sodium hydroxide into the water.

7. After you have added all the sodium hydroxide, use the wooden spoon to stir the solution.

8. The solution will warm up as the sodium hydroxide dissolves into the water. Ensure all the sodium hydroxide has dissolved into the water. Continue to stir until there are no crystals floating in the solution. As the sodium hydroxide dissolves into the water, the solution will become very warm. Make sure it is out of reach of children & pets.

9. Set the lye solution in a safe place and get the oils ready.

Measuring and Mixing the Oils

Oil Mixture			
Olive Oil	Sunflower Oil	Palm Oil	Coconut Oil
150 grams / 5.3 oz	125 grams / 4.4 oz	175 grams / 6.2 oz	468 grams / 16.5 oz

1. Place the glass bowl on the scale and tare the weight, or re-zero the scale. Weigh 468 g or 16.5 oz of coconut oil into the glass bowl.

2. Re-zero the scale and weigh the 175 g or 6.2 oz of palm oil into the bowl containing the coconut oil.

3. Transfer the glass bowl with the solid coconut and palm oil to the microwave or bain-marie and heat just until melted.

4. In a large glass bowl, pour the olive oil in until you have 150 g or 5.3 oz.

5. Re-zero the scale and add 125 g or 4.4oz of the sunflower to the same bowl.

6. Add the melted palm and coconut oil to the larger glass bowl containing the sunflower and olive oil.

7. Stir all oils together well using either a hand blender or whisk. Your oils are now ready to go.

Mixing the Soap

1. Slowly pour the lye solution into the large bowl containing the oil mixture. Stir slowly with a wooden spoon. If you prefer, you may stir with the stick mixture with the power off.

2.   After all the lye has been added and mixed with the oils, begin to stir with the stick mixer on. The oils and sodium hydroxide will start to react to produce soap and glycerin.

3.   Continue to stir using the stick mixer. The soap mixture will become more opaque and begin to thicken. You will notice the soap mixture will become more and more like a batter.

4.   Stir until the soap mixture is like a cake batter. At this point the soap will trace, or leave a pattern if drizzled over the surface. The soap is now ready to pour into the soap mould or pan.

Pouring the Soap

1.   Once the soap mixture has thickened and is at "trace", it is time to pour the soap mixture into the mould or pan.

2.   Slowly pour the soap into the pan. You may use a spatula to scrape the sides of the bowl.

3.   Gently tilt the pan to distribute the soap mixture until it is even in the pan.

4.   Wrap the soap with cling film and cover the soap with layers of towels to keep the heat in.

Soap Processing

1.   The soap will continue to process while it is wrapped in the towels. The chemical reaction will continue to produce soap and glycerine from the oil

2.   As the chemical reaction occurs and the soap heats further, the soap will enter a "gel" phase. If you peek at the soap you will notice the soap becoming more transparent and darker in the centre. The "gel" spreads to the edge of the pan as the chemical reaction occurs.

3.   Once the "gel" has reached the edge, you may unwrap the soap. At this point, there is minimal sodium hydroxide remaining in the soap. You can leave the soap wrapped until it has cooled completely if you prefer.

Finishing the Soap

1.   When the soap has cooled, remove the soap from the pan or tray.

2.   Cut immediately into pieces. If you wait to cut the soap, it may break when you cut it.

3.   Check pH of the finished soap. It will probably be about pH 9. When the soap below pH 10 is safe to use.

Basic Recipe 2- Olive, Sunflower & Palm Oil

The combination of olive, sunflower and palm oil gives a nice soap. The omission of coconut oil yields a soap with less lather but the combination of olive and sunflower adds an emollient quality to the soap.

Equipment
Scales
Rubber gloves
Large glass jar or a Pyrex measuring cup
Small plastic or glass bowl
Large glass bowl
Pan (9x9 inch)
Wooden spoon
Electric stick mixer
Microwave oven or bain-marie
Cling film
Towels
Spatula

Ingredients
125 g or 4.4 oz Sodium hydroxide (NaOH)
225 g / 7.9 oz Water
300 g / 10.6 oz Olive oil
200 g / 7.1 oz Sunflower oil
500 g / 17.6 oz Palm oil

Making the Lye Solution

Lye Solution	
Water	Sodium Hydroxide (NaOH)
225 grams / 7.9 oz	125 grams / 4.4 oz
Safety Advice: Always add sodium hydroxide to water!	

1. Place the large glass jar or Pyrex cup on the scale and re-zero the scale to eliminate the jar weight or note the weight of the jar.
2. Weigh the water into the jar so the water weight is 225 g or 7.9 oz.
3. Put the jar of water to the side and put on your gloves.
4. Place the small bowl on the scale and tare out the weight of the bowl. Carefully pour the sodium hydroxide into the bowl until you have 125 g or 4.4oz of sodium hydroxide.
5. Move to sink and place water jar in the sink. Slowly pour the sodium hydroxide into the large jar containing the water. You can swirl the jar to begin mixing the sodium hydroxide into the water.
6. After you have added all the sodium hydroxide, use the wooden spoon to stir the solution.

7. Ensure all the sodium hydroxide has dissolved into the water. Continue to stir until there are no crystals floating in the solution. The solution will warm up as the sodium hydroxide dissolves into the water. Make sure the lye solution is out of reach of children & pets.
8. Set the lye solution in a safe place and get the oils ready.

Measuring and Mixing the Oils

Oil Mixture		
Olive Oil	Sunflower Oil	Palm Oil
300 grams / 10.6 oz	200 grams / 7.1 oz	500 grams / 17.6 oz

1. Place the glass bowl on the scale and zero the scale. Weigh 500 g or 17.6 oz of palm oil into the glass bowl.
2. Put the palm oil to the microwave or bain-marie and heat just until melted.
3. Weigh 300 g or 10.6 oz olive oil into a large glass bowl. Re-zero the scale and add 200 g or 7.1 oz sunflower oil to the same bowl.
4. Add the melted palm oil to the larger glass bowl containing the sunflower and olive oil.
5. Stir all oils together well using either a hand blender or spoon. Your oils are now ready to go.

Mixing the Soap

1. Slowly pour the lye solution into the large bowl containing the oil mixture. Stir slowly with a wooden spoon. If you prefer, you may stir with the stick mixture with the power off.
2. After all the lye has been added and mixed with the oils, begin to stir with the stick mixer on. The oils and sodium hydroxide will start to react to produce soap and glycerin.
3. Continue to stir using the stick mixer. The soap mixture will become more opaque and begin to thicken. You will notice the soap mixture will become more and more like a batter.
4. Stir until the soap mixture is like a cake batter. At this point the soap will trace, or leave a pattern if drizzled over the surface. The soap is now ready to pour into the soap mould or pan.

Pouring the Soap

1. Once the soap mixture has thickened and is at "trace", it is time to pour the soap mixture into the mould or pan.
2. Slowly pour the soap into the pan. You may use a spatula to scrape the sides of the bowl.
3. Gently tilt the pan to distribute the soap mixture until it is even in the pan.
4. Wrap the soap with cling film and cover the soap with layers of towels to keep the heat in.

Soap Processing

1. The soap will continue to process while it is wrapped in the towels. The chemical reaction will continue to produce soap and glycerine from the oil
2. As the chemical reaction occurs and the soap heats further, the soap will enter a "gel" phase. If you peek at the soap you will notice the soap becoming more transparent and darker in the centre. The "gel" spreads to the edge of the pan as the chemical reaction occurs.
3. Once the "gel" has reached the edge, you may unwrap the soap. At this point, there is minimal sodium hydroxide remaining in the soap. You can leave the soap wrapped until it has cooled completely if you prefer.

Finishing the Soap

1. When the soap has cooled, remove the soap from the pan or tray.
2. Cut immediately into pieces. If you wait to cut the soap, it may break when you cut it.
3. Check pH of the finished soap. It will probably be about pH 9. Soap is below pH 10 it safe to use.

Basic Recipe 3- Olive, Coconut & Palm Oil

Palm oil makes this soap hard, coconut makes it bubble and olive oil adds moisture, a very good combination indeed.

Equipment
Scales
Rubber gloves
Large glass Jar or a Pyrex measuring cup
Small plastic or glass bowl
Large glass bowl

Ingredients
103 g / 3.6 oz Sodium hydroxide (NaOH)
190 g / 6.7 oz Water
200 g / 7.1 oz Olive oil
200 g / 7.1 oz Coconut oil
400 g / 14 oz Palm oil

Pan (9×9 inch)
Wooden spoon
Electric stick mixer
Microwave oven or bain-marie
Cling film
Towels

Making the Lye Solution

Lye Solution	
Water	Sodium Hydroxide (NaOH)
190 grams / 6.7 oz	103 grams / 3.6 oz
Safety Advice: Always add sodium hydroxide to water!	

1. Put on your gloves before making the lye solution.
2. Place the Pyrex measuring cup or large glass jar on the scale and zero the scale.
3. Pour the water into the jar until the weight is 190 g or 6.7 oz.
4. Put the jar of water to the side.
5. Place the small plastic or glass bowl on the scale and tare out the weight of the bowl. Carefully pour the sodium hydroxide into the bowl until you have 103 grams or 3.6 oz.
6. Move to sink and place water jar in the sink. Slowly pour the sodium hydroxide into the large jar containing the water.
7. After you have added all the sodium hydroxide, use the wooden spoon to stir the solution.
8. Ensure all the sodium hydroxide has dissolved. Continue to stir until there are no crystals floating in the solution. Keep the hot lye solution away from children & pets.
9. Set the lye solution in a safe place and get the oils ready.

Measuring and Mixing the Oils

Oil Mixture		
Olive Oil	Coconut Oil	Palm Oil
200 grams / 7.1 oz	200 grams / 7.1 oz	400 grams / 14 oz

1. Place the glass bowl on the scale, zero the scale and weigh 400 g or 14 oz of palm oil into the glass bowl.
2. Zero the scale again and weigh the 200 g or 7.1 oz of coconut oil into the bowl containing the palm oil.
3. Move the glass bowl with the solid coconut and palm oil to the microwave or bain-marie and heat until melted.
4. In a large glass bowl, pour the olive oil in until you have 200 g or 7.1 oz.
5. Add the melted palm and coconut oil to the larger glass bowl containing the olive oil.
6. Stir all oils together well using either a hand blender or whisk. Your oils are now ready to go.

Mixing the Soap

1. Slowly pour the lye solution into the large bowl containing the oil mixture. Stir slowly with a wooden spoon. If you prefer, you may stir with the stick mixture with the power off.
2. After all the lye has been added and mixed with the oils, begin to stir with the stick mixer on. The oils and sodium hydroxide will start to react to produce soap and glycerin.
3. Continue to stir using the stick mixer. The soap mixture will become more opaque and begin to thicken. You will notice the soap mixture will become more and more like a batter.
4. Stir until the soap mixture is like a cake batter. At this point the soap will trace, or leave a pattern if drizzled over the surface. The soap is now ready to pour into the soap mould or pan.

Pouring the Soap

1. Once the soap mixture has thickened and is at "trace", it is time to pour the soap mixture into the mould or pan.

2. Slowly pour the soap into the pan. You may use a spatula to scrape the sides.
3. Gently tilt the pan to distribute the soap mixture until it is even in the pan.
4. Wrap the soap with cling film and cover the soap with layers of towels to keep the heat in.

Soap Processing

1. The soap will continue to process while it is wrapped in the towels. The chemical reaction will continue to produce soap and glycerine from the oil
2. As the chemical reaction occurs and the soap heats further, the soap will enter a "gel" phase. If you peek at the soap you will notice the soap becoming more transparent and darker in the centre. The "gel" spreads to the edge of the pan as the chemical reaction occurs.
3. Once the "gel" has reached the edge, you may unwrap the soap. At this point, there is minimal sodium hydroxide remaining in the soap. You can leave the soap wrapped until it has cooled completely if you prefer.

Finishing the Soap

1. When the soap has cooled, remove the soap from the pan or tray.
2. Cut immediately into pieces. If you wait to cut the soap, it may break when you cut it.
3. Check pH of the finished soap. It will probably be about pH 9. Soap below pH 10 is safe to use.

Basic Recipe 4- Olive & Palm Oil

A traditional combination of olive and palm oil gives a very hard bar. Olive oil makes this soap very moisturising.

Equipment	*Ingredients*
Scales	117 g / 4.1 oz Sodium hydroxide
Rubber gloves	(NaOH)
Large glass jar or a Pyrex measuring cup	210 g / 7.4 oz Water
Small plastic or glass bowl	368 g / 13 oz Olive oil
Large glass bowl	550 g / 19.4 oz Palm oil
Pan (9x9 inch)	
Wooden Spoon	
Electric stick mixer	

Microwave oven or bain-Marie
Cling film
Towels

Making the Lye Solution

Lye Solution	
Water	Sodium Hydroxide (NaOH)
210 grams / 7.4 oz	117 grams / 4.1 oz
Safety Advice: Always add sodium hydroxide to water!	

1. Put on your gloves before you begin.
2. Put the Pyrex measuring cup or large glass jar on the scale. Zero the scale and weigh 210 g or 7.4 oz water.
3. Move the jar of water to the side.
4. Place the small bowl on the scale, tare out the weight and carefully pour the sodium hydroxide into the bowl until you have 117 g or 4.1 oz of sodium hydroxide.
5. Move to sink and place water jar in the sink. Slowly pour the sodium hydroxide into the large jar containing the water.
6. After you have added all the sodium hydroxide, use the wooden spoon to stir the sodium hydroxide. Ensure all the sodium hydroxide has dissolved into the water.
7. Set the lye solution in a safe place and get the oils ready.

Measuring and Mixing the Oils

Oil Mixture	
Olive Oil	Palm Oil
368 grams / 13 oz	550 grams / 19.4 oz

1. Place the large glass bowl on the scale and tare the weight, or re-zero the scale. Weigh 550 g or 19.4 oz of palm oil into the glass bowl.
2. Place the glass bowl of palm oil to the microwave or Bain-marie and heat until melted.
3. In another glass bowl, weigh the olive oil in until you have 368 g or 13 oz. Remember to zero the scale first.
4. Add the olive oil to the melted palm and stir. Your oils are now ready to go.

Mixing the Soap

1. Slowly pour the lye solution into the large bowl containing the oil mixture. Stir slowly with a wooden spoon. If you prefer, you may stir with the stick mixture with the power off.
2. After all the lye has been added and mixed with the oils, begin to stir with the stick mixer on. The oils and sodium hydroxide will start to react to produce soap and glycerin.
3. Continue to stir using the stick mixer. The soap mixture will become more opaque and begin to thicken. You will notice the soap mixture will become more and more like a batter.
4. Stir until the soap mixture is like a cake batter. At this point the soap will trace, or leave a pattern if drizzled over the surface. The soap is now ready to pour into the soap mould or pan.

Pouring the Soap

1. Once the soap mixture has thickened and is at "trace", it is time to pour the soap mixture into the mould or pan.
2. Slowly pour the soap into the pan. You may use a spatula to scrape the sides of the bowl.
3. Gently tilt the pan to distribute the soap mixture until it is even in the pan.
4. Wrap the soap with cling film and cover the soap with layers of towels to keep the heat in.

Soap Processing

1. The soap will continue to process while it is wrapped in the towels. The chemical reaction will continue to produce soap and glycerine from the oil
2. As the chemical reaction occurs and the soap heats further, the soap will enter a "gel" phase. If you peek at the soap you will notice the soap becoming more transparent and darker in the centre. The "gel" spreads to the edge of the pan as the chemical reaction occurs.
3. Once the "gel" has reached the edge, you may unwrap the soap. At this point, there is minimal sodium hydroxide remaining in the soap. You can leave the soap wrapped until it has cooled completely if you prefer.

Finishing the Soap

1. When the soap has cooled, remove the soap from the pan or tray.

2. Cut immediately into pieces. If you wait to cut the soap, it may break when you cut it.

3. Check pH of the finished soap. It will probably be about pH 9. Soap below pH 10 is safe to use.

Basic Recipe 5- Olive, Sweet Almond Oil & Vegetable Shortening

Vegetable shortening is a good option for those who wish to avoid palm oil. Shortening also makes soap hard, similar to palm oil. The combination of olive and sweet almond oil makes this soap moisturising. The lather of this bar is light.

Equipment	Ingredients
Scales	120 g / 4.2 oz Sodium hydroxide (NaOH)
Rubber gloves	
Large glass jar or a Pyrex measuring cup	215 g / 7.6 oz Water
Small plastic or glass bowl	300 g / 10.6 oz Olive oil
Large glass bowl	200 g / 7.1 oz Sweet Almond oil
Pan (9x9 inch)	450 g / 15.9 oz Vegetable shortening
Wooden spoon	
Electric stick mixer	
Microwave oven or bain-marie	
Cling film	
Towels	

Making the Lye Solution

Lye Solution	
Water	**Sodium Hydroxide (NaOH)**
215 grams / 7.6 oz	120 grams / 4.2 oz
Safety Advice: Always add sodium hydroxide to water!	

1. Wearing your gloves, place the large glass jar or Pyrex measuring cup on the scale. Zero the scale and weigh the water into the jar so the water weight is 215 g or 7.6 oz.

2. Place the small plastic or glass bowl on the scale, zero the scale and carefully weigh 120 g or 4.2 oz sodium hydroxide into the bowl.

3. Move to sink and place water jar in the sink. Slowly pour the sodium hydroxide into the large jar containing the water.

4. After you have added all the sodium hydroxide, stir with a wooden spoon.

5. Continue to stir until all the sodium hydroxide has dissolved into the water. Continue to stir until there are no crystals floating in the solution.
6. Set the lye solution in a safe place and get the oils ready.

Measuring and Mixing the Oils

Oil Mixture		
Olive Oil	Sweet Almond Oil	Veg. Shortening
300 grams / 10.6 oz	200 grams / 7.1 oz	450 grams / 15.9 oz

1. Place the glass bowl on the scale and tare the weight. Weigh 450 g or 15.9 oz of vegetable shortening into the glass bowl.
2. Transfer the glass bowl with the vegetable shortening to the microwave or bain-marie and melt.
3. Zero the scale and weigh the 300 g or 10.6 oz of olive oil
4. Re-zero the scale and add 200 g or 7.1 oz of the sweet almond oil into the same bowl.
5. Add the melted vegetable shortening to the larger glass bowl containing the sweet almond oil and olive oil.
6. Stir all oils together well using either a hand blender or spoon. Your oils are now ready to go.

Mixing the Soap

1. Slowly pour the lye solution into the large bowl containing the oil mixture. Stir slowly with a wooden spoon. If you prefer, you may stir with the stick mixture with the power off.
2. After all the lye has been added and mixed with the oils, begin to stir with the stick mixer on. The oils and sodium hydroxide will start to react to produce soap and glycerin.
3. Continue to stir using the stick mixer. The soap mixture will become more opaque and begin to thicken. You will notice the soap mixture will become more and more like a batter.
4. Stir until the soap mixture is like a cake batter. At this point the soap will trace, or leave a pattern if drizzled over the surface. The soap is now ready to pour into the soap mould or pan.

Pouring the Soap

1. Once the soap mixture has thickened and is at "trace", it is time to pour the soap mixture into the mould or pan.
2. Slowly pour the soap into the pan. You may use a spatula to scrape the sides of the bowl.
3. Gently tilt the pan to distribute the soap mixture until it is even in the pan.
4. Wrap the soap with cling film and cover the soap with layers of towels to keep the heat in.

Soap Processing

1. The soap will continue to process while it is wrapped in the towels. The chemical reaction will continue to produce soap and glycerine from the oil
2. As the chemical reaction occurs and the soap heats further, the soap will enter a "gel" phase. If you peek at the soap you will notice the soap becoming more transparent and darker in the centre. The "gel" spreads to the edge of the pan as the chemical reaction occurs.
3. Once the "gel" has reached the edge, you may unwrap the soap. At this point, there is minimal sodium hydroxide remaining in the soap. You can leave the soap wrapped until it has cooled completely if you prefer.

Finishing the Soap

1. When the soap has cooled, remove the soap from the pan or tray.
2. Cut immediately into pieces. If you wait to cut the soap, it may break when you cut it.
3. Check pH of the finished soap. It will probably be about pH 9. Soap below pH 10 is safe to use.

Basic Recipe 6- Castor, Coconut, Olive, & Palm

This soap has the addition of caster oil. The combination of caster oil and coconut oil give this soap superior lather. Also, caster oil and olive work together to yield high moisture.

Equipment	Ingredients
Scales	135 g / 4.8 oz Sodium hydroxide
Rubber gloves	(NaOH)
Large glass jar or a Pyrex measuring cup	245 g / 8.6 oz Water
Small plastic or glass bowl	100 g / 3.5 oz Castor oil
Large glass bowl	250 g / 8.8 oz Olive oil
Pan (9x9 inch)	250 g / 8.8 oz Coconut oil
Wooden spoon	400 g / 14 oz Palm oil
Electric stick mixer	
Microwave oven or bain-marie	
Cling film	
Towels	

Making the Lye Solution

Lye Solution	
Water	Sodium Hydroxide (NaOH)
245 grams / 8.6 oz	135 grams / 4.8 oz
Safety Advice: Always add sodium hydroxide to water!	

1. Put on your gloves
2. Place the large glass jar on the scale and zero the scale to eliminate the jar weight of the jar.
3. Weigh the water into the jar so the water weight is 245 g or 8.6 oz.
4. Put the jar of water to the side.
5. Place the small plastic or glass bowl on the scale and tare out the weight of the bowl or re-zero the scale. Carefully pour the sodium hydroxide into the bowl until you have 135 g or 4.8oz of sodium hydroxide.
6. Move to sink and place water jar in the sink. Slowly pour the sodium hydroxide into the large jar containing the water. You can swirl the jar to begin mixing the sodium hydroxide into the water.
7. After you have added all the sodium hydroxide, use the wooden spoon to stir the sodium hydroxide. You may wish to have a dedicated spoon for mixing lye, rather than a spoon contaminated with "cooking odour". The odour might transfer

from the spoon to your lye and into your soap. In my opinion, onion-scented soap is not very desirable.

8. The solution will warm up as the sodium hydroxide dissolves into the water. Ensure all the sodium hydroxide has dissolved into the water. Continue to stir until there are no crystals floating in the solution. Make sure it is out of reach of children & pets.

9. Set the lye solution in a safe place and get the oils ready.

Measuring and Mixing the Oils

It is necessary that the oils be measured by weight. Be sure you have enough of each oil. When weighing water, 500 ml weighs 500 grams, so a 500 ml bottle gives you 500 grams of water. Oil weighs less than water and so a 500 ml bottle will be less than 500 g. Many oils in are available in 250 ml bottles. Again, 250 ml will not give you 250 g. You will need to buy two, 250 ml bottles.

Oil Mixture			
Castor	Olive Oil	Palm Oil	Coconut Oil
100 grams / 3.5 oz	250 grams / 8.8 oz	400 grams / 14 oz	250 grams / 8.8 oz

1. Gather the following: oils, scale, plastic container, microwave safe bowl (if the plastic container is microwave safe, you can use this), and Electric stick mixer

2. Place the glass bowl on the scale and tare the weight, or re-zero the scale. Weigh 250 g or 8.8 oz of coconut oil into the glass jar.

3. Re-zero the scale and weigh the 400 g or 14 oz of palm oil into the bowl containing the coconut oil.

4. Transfer the glass bowl with the solid coconut and palm oil to the microwave or bain-marie and heat just until melted.

5. In a large glass bowl, pour the olive oil in until you have 250 g or 8.8 oz.

6. Re-zero the scale and add 100 g or 3.5 oz of castor oil to the same bowl.

7. Add the melted palm and coconut oil to the larger glass bowl containing the castor and olive oil.

8. Stir all oils together well using either a hand blender or spoon. Your oils are now ready to go.

Mixing the Soap

1. Slowly pour the lye solution into the large bowl containing the oil mixture. Stir slowly with a wooden spoon. If you prefer, you may stir with the stick mixture with the power off.
2. After all the lye has been added and mixed with the oils, begin to stir with the stick mixer on. The oils and sodium hydroxide will start to react to produce soap and glycerin.
3. Continue to stir using the stick mixer. The soap mixture will become more opaque and begin to thicken. You will notice the soap mixture will become more and more like a batter.
4. Stir until the soap mixture is like a cake batter. At this point the soap will trace, or leave a pattern if drizzled over the surface. The soap is now ready to pour into the soap mould or pan.

Pouring the Soap

1. Once the soap mixture has thickened and is at "trace", it is time to pour the soap mixture into the mould or pan.
2. Slowly pour the soap into the pan. You may use a spatula to scrape the sides.
3. Gently tilt the pan to distribute the soap mixture until it is even in the pan.
4. Wrap the soap with cling film and cover the soap with layers of towels to keep the heat in.

Soap Processing

1. The soap will continue to process while it is wrapped in the towels. The chemical reaction will continue to produce soap and glycerine from the oil
2. As the chemical reaction occurs and the soap heats further, the soap will enter a "gel" phase. If you peek at the soap you will notice the soap becoming more transparent and darker in the centre. The "gel" spreads to the edge of the pan as the chemical reaction occurs.
3. Once the "gel" has reached the edge, you may unwrap the soap. At this point, there is minimal sodium hydroxide remaining in the soap. You can leave the soap wrapped until it has cooled completely if you prefer.

Finishing the Soap

1. When the soap has cooled, remove the soap from the pan or tray.
2. Cut immediately into pieces. If you wait to cut the soap, it may break when you cut it.
3. Check pH of the finished soap. It will probably be about pH 9. Soap below pH 10 is safe to use.

Chapter 11

Honey Soap Recipes

Soap recipes can be divided into two parts, the fixed part consisting of the oils and sodium hydroxide involved in the saponification chemistry and the flexible part or the additional ingredients. The basic soaps recipes are examples of the fixed portion of the soap recipe. To each of the basic recipes you can add any additives, this is the flexible part of a recipe. The following recipes are composed of both a fixed and flexible section. When you read these recipes, you will see the fixed section of the recipe is the part consisting of the lye solution and oil mixture. These are the two reactants in the chemical reaction which makes the soap. The flexible section of the recipe is the additive section. You may omit any of these ingredients or substitute a similar ingredient.

If we take a closer look at the first recipe, lavender chamomile honey soap, we can identify the fixed and flexible parts of the recipe. The fixed section is composed of the lye solution and the oil mixture. Therefore, the fixed ingredients are; sodium hydroxide, water, olive oil, sunflower oil, palm oil, and coconut oil. You must have these ingredients to make this recipe. All of these ingredients are necessary for soap formation. The other ingredients, the ingredients listed as additional ingredients comprise the flexible part of the recipe. These include; lavender honey, ultramarine purple, chamomile tea, lavender fragrance oil, and chamomile fragrance oil. If you have blossom honey and not lavender honey, you may substitute. Perhaps you do not want to add the chamomile tea. That is fine too. If you strip away the additional ingredients from any recipe, you are left with a base soap recipe.

Lavender Chamomile Honey Soap

Equipment	Ingredients
Scales	112 g / 4 oz Sodium Hydroxide (NaOH)
Rubber gloves	
Large glass jar or a Pyrex measuring cup	200 g / 7 oz Water
Small plastic or glass bowl	150 g / 5.3 oz Olive oil
Large glass bowl	125 g / 4.4 oz Sunflower oil
Pan (9x9 inch)	175 g / 6.2 oz Palm oil
Wooden spoon	468 g / 16.5 oz Coconut oil
Electric stick mixer	15 ml / 1 T Lavender honey
Microwave oven or bain-marie	1 tsp Ultramarine purple
Cling film	1 sachet / 1 T Chamomile tea
Towels	15 ml / 1 T Lavender fragrance oil
Measuring spoons, teaspoon, tablespoon	15 ml / 1 T Chamomile fragrance oil

Making the Lye Solution

Lye Solution	
Water	Sodium Hydroxide (NaOH)
200 grams / 7 oz	112 g / 4 oz
Safety Advice: Always add sodium hydroxide to water!	

1. Put on your gloves before you begin.
2. Place the large glass jar on the scale and zero the scale to eliminate the weight of the jar.
3. Weigh the water into the jar so the water weight is 200 g or 7 oz.
4. Place the small plastic or glass bowl on the scale and tare out the weight of the bowl or re-zero the scale. Carefully pour the sodium hydroxide into the bowl until you have 112 g or 4oz of sodium hydroxide.
5. Move to sink and place water jar in the sink. Slowly pour the sodium hydroxide into the large jar containing the water. You can swirl the jar to begin mixing the sodium hydroxide into the water.
6. After you have added all the sodium hydroxide, use the wooden spoon to stir the sodium hydroxide..

7. Ensure all the sodium hydroxide has dissolved into the water. Continue to stir until there are no crystals floating in the solution. The solution will warm up as the sodium hydroxide dissolves into the water. Make sure it is out of reach of children & pets.
8. Set the lye solution in a safe place and get the oils ready.

Measuring and Mixing the Oils

Oil Mixture			
Olive Oil	Sunflower Oil	Palm Oil	Coconut Oil
150 grams / 5.3 oz	125 grams / 4.4 oz	175 grams / 6.2 oz	468 grams / 16.5 oz

1. Place the glass bowl on the scale and tare the weight, or re-zero the scale. Weigh 468 g or 16.5 oz of coconut oil into the glass bowl.
2. Re-zero the scale and weigh the 175 g or 6.2 oz of palm oil into the bowl containing the coconut oil.
3. Transfer the glass bowl with the solid coconut and palm oil to the microwave or bain-marie and heat just until melted.
4. In a large glass bowl, pour the olive oil in until you have 150 g or 5.3 oz.
5. Re-zero the scale and add 125 g or 4.4 oz of the sunflower to the same bowl.
6. Add the melted palm and coconut oil to the larger glass bowl containing the sunflower and olive oil.
7. Stir all oils together well using either a hand blender or whisk. Your oils are now ready to go.

Additional Ingredients

Additional Ingredients			
Honey	Colour	Botanical	Fragrance Oils
Lavender	Ultramarine Purple	Chamomile Flowers	Lavender & Chamomile
15 ml or 1 T	1 tsp	1 sachet tea or 1 T	15 ml or 1 T each
add to oil mix	add to oil mix	add to oil mix	add at trace

1. Add 15 ml or 1 T lavender honey and 1 tsp ultramarine purple to the oil mixture and stir with the stick mixer until the ultramarine is dispersed.
2. Empty the contents of 1 sachet chamomile tea into the oil mix. Alternatively, add 1 T of loose chamomile tea. Stir.
3. Have the fragrance oils to hand. These will be added just prior to pouring the soap into the pan.

Mixing the Soap

1. Slowly pour the lye solution into the large bowl containing the oil mixture. Stir slowly with a wooden spoon. If you prefer, you may stir with the stick mixture with the power off.
2. After all the lye has been added and mixed with the oils, begin to stir with the stick mixer on. The oils and sodium hydroxide will start to react to produce soap and glycerin.
3. Continue to stir using the stick mixer. The soap mixture will become more opaque and begin to thicken. You will notice the soap mixture will become more and more like a batter.
4. Add the lavender and chamomile fragrance oil to the soap mixture and continue to stir.
5. Stir until the soap mixture is like a cake batter. At this point the soap will trace, or leave a pattern if drizzled over the surface. The soap is now ready to pour into the soap mould or pan.

Pouring the Soap

1. Once the soap mixture has thickened and is at "trace", it is time to pour the soap mixture into the mould or pan.
2. Slowly pour the soap into the pan. You may use a spatula to scrape the sides.
3. Gently tilt the pan to distribute the soap mixture until it is even in the pan.
4. Wrap the soap with cling film and cover the soap with layers of towels to keep the heat in.

Soap Processing

1. The soap will continue to process while it is wrapped in the towels. The chemical reaction will continue to produce soap and glycerine from the oil
2. As the chemical reaction occurs and the soap heats further, the soap will enter a "gel" phase. If you peek at the soap you will notice the soap becoming more transparent and darker in the centre. The "gel" spreads to the edge of the pan as

the chemical reaction occurs.

3. Once the "gel" has reached the edge, you may unwrap the soap. At this point, there is minimal sodium hydroxide remaining in the soap. You can leave the soap wrapped until it has cooled completely if you prefer.

Finishing the Soap

1. When the soap has cooled, remove the soap from the pan or tray.
2. Cut immediately into pieces. If you wait to cut the soap, it may break when you cut it.
3. Check pH of the finished soap. It will probably be about pH 9. Soap below pH 10 is safe to use.

Honey Bee Soap

Equipment	*Ingredients*
Scales	112 g / 4 oz Sodium hydroxide
Rubber gloves	(NaOH)
Large glass jar or a Pyrex measuring cup	200 g / 7 oz Water
Small plastic or glass bowl	150 g / 5.3 oz Olive oil
Large glass bowl	125 g / 4.4 oz Sunflower oil
Pan (9x9 inch)	175 g / 6.2 oz Palm oil
Wooden spoon	468 g / 16.5 oz Coconut oil
Electric stick mixer	15 ml / 1 T Blossom honey
Microwave oven or bain-marie	1/2 sheet natural beeswax (candle
Cling film	sheet)
Towels	90 ml/ 6 T Blossom honey
Measuring spoons, teaspoon, tablespoon	30 ml/ 2 T Mimosa fragrance oil

Making the Lye Solution

Lye Solution	
Water	Sodium Hydroxide (NaOH)
200 grams / 7 oz	112 g / 4 oz
Safety Advice: Always add sodium hydroxide to water!	

1. Before you begin, put on your gloves.
2. Place the large glass jar on the scale and zero the scale to eliminate the weight of the jar.
3. Weigh the water into the jar so the water weight is 200 g or 7 oz.
4. Place the small plastic or glass bowl on the scale and tare out the weight of the bowl or re-zero the scale. Carefully pour the sodium hydroxide into the bowl until you have 112 g or 4 oz of sodium hydroxide.
5. Move to sink and place water jar in the sink. Slowly pour the sodium hydroxide into the large jar containing the water. You can swirl the jar to begin mixing the sodium hydroxide into the water.
6. After you have added all the sodium hydroxide, use the wooden spoon to stir the sodium hydroxide. Stir slowly until all crystals have dissolved.
7. Set the lye solution in a safe place and get the oils ready.

Measuring and Mixing the Oils

Oil Mixture			
Olive Oil	Sunflower Oil	Palm Oil	Coconut Oil
150 grams / 5.3 oz	125 grams / 4.4 oz	175 grams / 6.2 oz	468 grams / 16.5 oz

1. Place the glass bowl on the scale and tare the weight, or re-zero the scale. Weigh 468 g or 16.5 oz of coconut oil into the glass jar.
2. Re-zero the scale and weigh the 175 g or 6.2 oz of palm oil into the bowl containing the coconut oil.
3. Transfer the glass bowl with the solid coconut and palm oil to the microwave or bain-marie and heat just until melted.
4. In a large glass bowl, pour the olive oil in until you have 150 g or 5.3 oz.
5. Re-zero the scale and add 125 g or 4.4 oz sunflower oil to the same bowl.
6. Add the melted palm and coconut oil to the larger glass bowl containing the sunflower and olive oil.
7. Stir all oils together well using either a hand blender or spoon. Your oils are now ready to go.

Additional Ingredients

Additional Ingredients			
Honey	Beeswax	Honey	Fragrance Oils
Blossom	Natural Sheet	Blossom	Mimosa
90 ml or 6 T	½ sheet torn into pieces	15 ml or 1 T	30 ml or 2 T
bottom of pan	bottom of pan	add to oil mix	add at trace

1. Tear the beeswax sheet into rough edged pieces approximately 1 x 1 inch. Stick the pieces onto the bottom of the 9 x 9 "pan leaving spaces between the pieces.
2. Spread the 90 ml or 6 T of honey into the spaces between the beeswax pattern. The honey and the beeswax will be on the top of the soap and will give the appearance of honeycomb.
3. Add 15 ml or 1 T blossom honey into to the oil mixture and stir.
4. Have the fragrance oils to hand. These will be added just prior to pouring the soap into the pan.

Mixing the Soap

1. Slowly pour the lye solution into the large bowl containing the oil mixture. Stir slowly with a wooden spoon. If you prefer, you may stir with the stick mixture with the power off.
2. After all the lye has been added and mixed with the oils, begin to stir with the stick mixer on. The oils and sodium hydroxide will start to react to produce soap and glycerin.
3. Continue to stir using the stick mixer. The soap mixture will become more opaque and begin to thicken. You will notice the soap mixture will become more and more like a batter.
4. Add the mimosa fragrance oil to the soap mixture and continue to stir.
5. Stir until the soap mixture is like a cake batter. At this point the soap will trace, or leave a pattern if drizzled over the surface. The soap is now ready to pour into the soap mould or pan.

Pouring the Soap

1. Once the soap mixture has thickened and is at "trace", it is time to pour the soap mixture into the mould or pan.
2. Slowly pour the soap into the pan. You may use a spatula to scrape the sides of the bowl.
3. Gently tilt the pan to distribute the soap mixture until it is even in the pan.
4. Wrap the soap with cling film and cover the soap with layers of towels to keep the heat in.

Soap Processing

1. The soap will continue to process while it is wrapped in the towels. The chemical reaction will continue to produce soap and glycerine from the oil
2. As the chemical reaction occurs and the soap heats further, the soap will enter a "gel" phase. If you peek at the soap you will notice the soap becoming more transparent and darker in the centre. The "gel" spreads to the edge of the pan as the chemical reaction occurs.
3. Once the "gel" has reached the edge, you may unwrap the soap. At this point, there is minimal sodium hydroxide remaining in the soap. You can leave the soap wrapped until it has cooled completely if you prefer.

Finishing the Soap

1. When the soap has cooled, remove the soap from the pan or tray.
2. Cut immediately into pieces. If you wait to cut the soap, it may break when you cut it.
3. Check pH of the finished soap. It will probably be about pH 9. Soap below pH 10 is safe to use.

Orange Blossom & Carrot Soap

Equipment
Scales
Rubber gloves
Large glass jar or a Pyrex measuring cup
Small plastic or glass bowl
Large glass bowl
Pan (9x9 inch)
Wooden Spoon
Electric stick mixer
Microwave oven or bain-marie
Cling film
Towels
Measuring spoons, teaspoon, tablespoon

Ingredients
125 g / 4.4 oz Sodium hydroxide
(NaOH)
225 g / 7.9 oz Water
300 g / 10.6 oz Olive oil
200 g / 7.1 oz Sunflower oil
500 g / 17.6 oz Palm oil
15 ml / 1 T Blossom honey
50g /1.8 oz Carrot oil
30 ml/ 2 T Orange fragrance oil
3 T French green clay

Making the Lye Solution

Lye Solution	
Water	Sodium Hydroxide (NaOH)
225 g / 7.9 oz	125 g / 4.4 oz
Safety Advice: Always add sodium hydroxide to water!	

1. Begin by putting on your gloves.
2. Place the large glass jar on the scale and re-zero the scale to eliminate the weight of the jar.
3. Weigh the water into the jar so the water weight is 225 g or 7.9 oz.
4. Place the small plastic or glass bowl on the scale and tare out the weight of the bowl or re-zero the scale. Carefully pour the sodium hydroxide into the bowl until you have 125 g or 4.4 oz of sodium hydroxide.
5. Move to sink and place water jar in the sink. Slowly pour the sodium hydroxide into the large jar containing the water. You can swirl the jar to begin mixing the sodium hydroxide into the water.
6. After you have added all the sodium hydroxide, use the wooden spoon to stir the sodium hydroxide. Ensure all the sodium hydroxide has dissolved into the water. Continue to stir until there are no crystals floating in the solution.
7. Set the lye solution in a safe place and get the oils ready.

Measuring and Mixing the Oils

Oil Mixture		
Olive Oil	Sunflower Oil	Palm Oil
300 grams / 10.6 oz	200 grams / 7.1 oz	500 grams / 17.6oz

1. Place the glass bowl on the scale and tare the weight, or re-zero the scale. Weigh 500 g or 17.6 oz of palm oil into the glass bowl.
2. Transfer the glass bowl with the palm oil to the microwave or bain-marie and heat just until melted.
3. In a large glass bowl, pour the olive oil in until you have 300 g or 10.6 oz.
4. Re-zero the scale and add 200 g or 7.1 oz of the sunflower to the same bowl.
5. Add the melted palm oil to the larger glass bowl containing the sunflower and olive oil.
6. Stir all oils together well using either a hand blender or spoon. Your oils are now ready to go.

Additional Ingredients

Additional Ingredients			
Honey	Oil	Fragrance	Clay
Blossom	Carrot Oil	Orange	French Green Clay
15 ml or 1 T	50 g or 1.8 oz	30 ml or 2 T	3 T
add to oil mix	add to oil mix	add at trace	sprinkle on top after pouring

1. Add 15 ml or 1 T blossom honey into to the oil mixture and stir.
2. Weight 50 g or 1.8 oz of carrot oil and add to oil mixture. Stir.
3. Have the fragrance oil and green clay to hand.

Mixing the Soap

1. Slowly pour the lye solution into the large bowl containing the oil mixture. Stir slowly with a wooden spoon. If you prefer, you may stir with the stick mixture with the power off.
2. After all the lye has been added and mixed with the oils, begin to stir with the stick mixer on. The oils and sodium hydroxide will start to react to produce soap and glycerin.
3. Continue to stir using the stick mixer. The soap mixture will become more opaque and begin to thicken. You will notice the soap mixture will become more and more like a batter.
4. Add the orange fragrance oil to the soap mixture and continue to stir.
5. Stir until the soap mixture is like a cake batter. At this point the soap will trace, or leave a pattern if drizzled over the surface. The soap is now ready to pour into the soap mould or pan.

Pouring the Soap

1. Once the soap mixture has thickened and is at "trace", it is time to pour the soap mixture into the mould or pan.
2. Slowly pour the soap into the pan. You may use a spatula to scrape the bowl's sides.
3. Gently tilt the pan to distribute the soap mixture until it is even in the pan.
4. Sprinkle the top of the soap with the French green clay.
5. Wrap the soap with cling film and cover the soap with layers of towels to keep the heat in.

Soap Processing

1. The soap will continue to process while it is wrapped in the towels. The chemical reaction will continue to produce soap and glycerine from the oil
2. As the chemical reaction occurs and the soap heats further, the soap will enter a "gel" phase. If you peak at the soap you will notice the soap becoming more transparent and darker in the centre. The "gel" spreads to the edge of the pan as the chemical reaction occurs.
3. Once the "gel" has reached the edge, you may unwrap the soap. At this point, there is minimal sodium hydroxide remaining in the soap. You can leave the soap wrapped until it has cooled completely if you prefer.

Finishing the Soap

1. When the soap has cooled, remove the soap from the pan or tray.
2. Cut immediately into pieces. If you wait to cut the soap, it may break when you cut it.
3. Check pH of the finished soap. It will probably be about pH 9. Soap below pH 10 is safe to use.

Cocoa Island Soap

Equipment
Scales
Rubber gloves
Large glass jar or a Pyrex measuring cup
Small plastic or glass bowl
Large glass bowl
Pan (9x9 inch)
Wooden spoon
Electric stick mixer
Microwave oven or bain-marie
Cling film
Towels
Measuring spoons, teaspoon, tablespoon

Ingredients
103 g / 3.6 oz Sodium hydroxide (NaOH)
190 g / 6.7 oz Water
200 g / 7.1 oz Olive oil
200 g / 7.1 oz Coconut oil
400 g / 14 oz Palm oil
50 g / 1.8 oz Cocoa butter chips
15 ml /1 T Blossom honey
30 ml/ 2 T Coconut fragrance oil

Making the Lye Solution

Lye Solution	
Water	Sodium Hydroxide (NaOH)
190 grams / 6.7 oz	103 grams / 3.6 oz
Safety Advice: Always add sodium hydroxide to water!	

1. Put on your gloves.
2. Place the large glass jar on the scale and re-zero the scale to eliminate the weight of the jar.
3. Weigh the water into the jar so the water weight is 190 g or 6.7 oz.
4. Place the small plastic or glass bowl on the scale and tare out the weight of the bowl or re-zero the scale. Carefully pour the sodium hydroxide into the bowl

until you have 103 g or 3.6 oz of sodium hydroxide.

5. Move to sink and place water jar in the sink. Slowly pour the sodium hydroxide into the large jar containing the water.
6. After you have added all the sodium hydroxide, use the wooden spoon to stir the sodium hydroxide. Continue to stir until there are no crystals floating in the solution.
7. Set the lye solution in a safe place and get the oils ready.

Measuring and Mixing the Oils

Oil Mixture		
Olive Oil	Coconut Oil	Palm Oil
200 g / 7.1 oz	200 g / 7.1 oz	400 g / 14 oz

1. Place the glass bowl on the scale and tare the weight, or re-zero the scale. Weigh 200 g or 7.1 oz of coconut oil into the glass bowl.
2. Re-zero the scale and weigh the 400 g or 14 oz of palm oil into the bowl containing the coconut oil.
3. Transfer the glass bowl with the solid coconut and palm oil to the microwave or bain-marie and heat just until melted.
4. In a large glass bowl, pour the olive oil in until you have 200 g or 7.1 oz.
5. Add the melted palm and coconut oil to the larger glass bowl containing the olive oil.
6. Stir all oils together well using either a hand blender or whisk. Your oils are now ready to go.

Additional Ingredients

Additional Ingredients		
Honey	Fragrance Oil	Oil
Blossom	Coconut	Cocoa Butter Chips
15 ml or 1 T	30 ml or 2 T	50 g or 1.8 oz
add to oil mix	add at trace	sprinkle over soap in pan

1. Add 15 ml or 1 T blossom honey into to the oil mixture and stir.
2. Have the fragrance oil and cocoa butter chips to hand.

Mixing the Soap

1. Slowly pour the lye solution into the large bowl containing the oil mixture. Stir slowly with a wooden spoon. If you prefer, you may stir with the stick mixture with the power off.
2. After all the lye has been added and mixed with the oils, begin to stir with the stick mixer on. The oils and sodium hydroxide will start to react to produce soap and glycerin.
3. Continue to stir using the stick mixer. The soap mixture will become more opaque and begin to thicken. You will notice the soap mixture will become more and more like a batter.
4. Add the coconut oil to the soap mixture and continue to stir.
5. Stir until the soap mixture is like a cake batter. At this point the soap will trace, or leave a pattern if drizzled over the surface. The soap is now ready to pour into the soap mould or pan.

Pouring the Soap

1. Once the soap mixture has thickened and is at "trace", it is time to pour the soap mixture into the mould or pan.
2. Slowly pour the soap into the pan. You may use a spatula to scrape the sides.
3. Gently tilt the pan to distribute the soap mixture until it is even in the pan.
4. Sprinkle the cocoa butter chips over the top. If will fall into the soap and give the soap areas where there is unsaponified cocoa butter.
5. Wrap the soap with cling film and cover the soap with layers of towels to keep the heat in.

Soap Processing

1. The soap will continue to process while it is wrapped in the towels. The chemical reaction will continue to produce soap and glycerine from the oil
2. As the chemical reaction occurs and the soap heats further, the soap will enter a "gel" phase. If you peek at the soap you will notice the soap becoming more transparent and darker in the centre. The "gel" spreads to the edge of the pan as the chemical reaction occurs.

3. Once the "gel" has reached the edge, you may unwrap the soap. At this point, there is minimal sodium hydroxide remaining in the soap. You can leave the soap wrapped until it has cooled completely if you prefer.

Finishing the Soap

1. When the soap has cooled, remove the soap from the pan or tray. Make sure the soap is cooled completely or the cocoa butter will run.
2. Cut immediately into pieces. If you wait to cut the soap, it may break when you cut it.
3. Check pH of the finished soap. It will probably be about pH 9. Soap below pH 10 is safe to use.

Pink Lemonade Soap

Equipment	*Ingredients*
Scales	112 g / 4 oz Sodium hydroxide
Rubber gloves	(NaOH)
Large glass jar or a Pyrex measuring cup	200 g / 7 oz Water
Small plastic or glass bowl	150 g / 5.3 oz Olive oil
Large glass bowl	125 g / 4.4 oz Sunflower oil
Pan (9x9 inch)	175 g / 6.2 oz Palm oil
Wooden spoon	468 g / 16.5 oz Coconut oil
Electric stick mixer	15 ml / 1 T Lavender honey
Microwave oven or bain-marie	1 tsp Ultramarine pink
Cling film	15 ml / 1 T Lavender fragrance oil
Towels	15 ml / 1 T Lemon fragrance oil
Measuring spoons, teaspoon, tablespoon	

Making the Lye Solution

Lye Solution	
Water	**Sodium Hydroxide (NaOH)**
200 grams / 7 oz	112 g / 4 oz
Safety Advice: Always add sodium hydroxide to water!	

1. Begin by putting on your gloves.
2. Place the large glass jar on the scale and re-zero the scale to eliminate the weight of the jar.
3. Weigh the water into the jar so the water weight is 200 g or 7 oz.
4. Place the small plastic or glass bowl on the scale and tare out the weight of the bowl or re-zero the scale. Carefully pour the sodium hydroxide into the bowl until you have 112 g or 4oz of sodium hydroxide.
5. Move to sink and place water jar in the sink. Slowly pour the sodium hydroxide into the large jar containing the water. You can swirl the jar to begin mixing the sodium hydroxide into the water.
6. After you have added all the sodium hydroxide, use the wooden spoon to stir the sodium hydroxide. The solution will warm up as the sodium hydroxide dissolves into the water. Ensure all the sodium hydroxide has dissolved into the water.
7. Set the lye solution in a safe place and get the oils ready.

Measuring and Mixing the Oils

Oil Mixture			
Olive Oil	Sunflower Oil	Palm Oil	Coconut Oil
150 grams / 5.3 oz	125 grams / 4.4 oz	175 grams / 6.2 oz	468 grams / 16.5 oz

1. Place the glass bowl on the scale and tare the weight, or re-zero the scale. Weigh 468 g or 16.5 oz of coconut oil into the glass jar.
2. Re-zero the scale and weigh the 175 g or 6.2 oz of palm oil into the bowl containing the coconut oil.
3. Transfer the glass bowl with the solid coconut and palm oil to the microwave or Bain-marie and heat just until melted.
4. In a large glass bowl, pour the olive oil in until you have 150 g or 5.3 oz.
5. Re-zero the scale and add 125 g or 4.4 oz of the sunflower oil into the same bowl.
6. Add the melted palm and coconut oil to the larger glass bowl containing the sunflower and olive oil.
7. Stir all oils together well using either a hand blender or whisk. Your oils are now ready to go.

Additional Ingredients

Additional Ingredients		
Honey	Colour	Fragrance Oil
Lavender	Ultramine Pink	Lavender & Lemon
15 ml or 1 T	1 tsp	15 ml or 1 T each
add to oil mix	add to oil mix	add at trace

1. Add 15 ml or 1 T lavender honey and 1 tsp ultramarine pink into the oil mixture and stir with the stick mixer until the ultramarine is dispersed.
2. Have the fragrance oils to hand. These will be added just prior to pouring the soap into the pan.

Mixing the Soap

1. Slowly pour the lye solution into the large bowl containing the oil mixture. Stir slowly with a wooden spoon. If you prefer, you may stir with the stick mixture with the power off.
2. After all the lye has been added and mixed with the oils, begin to stir with the stick mixer on. The oils and sodium hydroxide will start to react to produce soap and glycerin.
3. Continue to stir using the stick mixer. The soap mixture will become more opaque and begin to thicken. You will notice the soap mixture will become more and more like a batter.
4. Add the lavender and lemon fragrance oil to the soap mixture and continue to stir.
5. Stir until the soap mixture is like a cake batter. At this point the soap will trace, or leave a pattern if drizzled over the surface. The soap is now ready to pour into the soap mould or pan.

Pouring the Soap

1. Once the soap mixture has thickened and is at "trace", it is time to pour the soap mixture into the mould or pan.
2. Slowly pour the soap into the pan. You may use a spatula to scrape the sides.
3. Gently tilt the pan to distribute the soap mixture until it is even in the pan.
4. Wrap the soap with cling film and cover the soap with layers of towels to keep the heat in.

Soap Processing

1. The soap will continue to process while it is wrapped in the towels. The chemical reaction will continue to produce soap and glycerine from the oil
2. As the chemical reaction occurs and the soap heats further, the soap will enter a "gel" phase. If you peek at the soap you will notice the soap becoming more transparent and darker in the centre. The "gel" spreads to the edge of the pan as the chemical reaction occurs.
3. Once the "gel" has reached the edge, you may unwrap the soap. At this point, there is minimal sodium hydroxide remaining in the soap. You can leave the soap wrapped until it has cooled completely if you prefer.

Finishing the Soap

1. When the soap has cooled, remove the soap from the pan or tray.
2. Cut immediately into pieces. If you wait to cut the soap, it may break when you cut it.
3. Check pH of the finished soap. It will probably be about pH 9. Soap below pH 10 is safe to use.

Green Earth Soap

Equipment
Scales
Rubber gloves
Large glass jar or a Pyrex measuring cup
Small plastic or glass bowl
Large glass bowl
Pan (9x9 inch)
Wooden spoon
Electric stick mixer
Microwave oven or bain-marie
Cling film
Towels

Ingredients
125 g / 4.4 oz Sodium hydroxide (NaOH)
225 g / 7.9 oz Water
300 g / 10.6 oz Olive oil
200 g / 7.1 oz Sunflower oil
500 g / 17.6 oz Palm oil
6 T French green clay
15 ml / 1 T Ivy honey
30 ml/ 2 T Ivy fragrance oil

Making the Lye Solution

Lye Solution	
Water	Sodium Hydroxide (NaOH)
225 grams / 7.9 oz	125 grams / 4.4 oz
Safety Advice: Always add sodium hydroxide to water!	

1. Put on your gloves before you start.
2. Place the large glass jar on the scale and zero the scale to eliminate the weight of the jar.
3. Weigh the water into the jar so the water weight is 225 g or 7.9 oz.
4. Place the small plastic or glass bowl on the scale and tare out the weight of the bowl. Carefully pour the sodium hydroxide into the bowl until you have 125 g or 4.4 oz of sodium hydroxide.
5. Move to sink and place water jar in the sink. Slowly pour the sodium hydroxide into the large jar containing the water
6. After you have added all the sodium hydroxide, use the wooden spoon to stir the sodium hydroxide.
7. Set the lye solution in a safe place and get the oils ready.

Measuring and Mixing the Oils

2. Oil Mixture		
Olive Oil	Sunflower Oil	Palm Oil
300 grams / 10.6 oz	200 grams / 7.1 oz	500 grams / 17.6 oz

1. Place the glass bowl on the scale and tare the weight, or re-zero the scale. Weigh 500 g or 17.6 oz of palm oil into the glass jar.
2. Transfer the glass bowl with the solid palm oil to the microwave or bain-marie and heat just until melted.
3. In a large glass bowl, pour the olive oil in until you have 300 g or 10.6 oz.
4. Re-zero the scale and add 200 g or 7.1 oz of the sunflower oil into the same bowl.
5. Add the melted palm oil to the larger glass bowl containing the sunflower and olive oil.
6. Stir all oils together well using either a hand blender or spoon. Your oils are now ready to go.

Additional Ingredients

Additional Ingredients			
Honey	**Clay**	**Fragrance Oil**	**Clay**
Ivy	French Green Clay	Ivy	French Green Clay
15 ml or 1 T	1 T	30 ml or 2 T	5 T
add to oil mix	add to oil mix	add at trace	sprinkle on top after pouring

1. Add 15 ml or 1 T Ivy honey and 1 T French green clay to the oil mixture and stir with the stick mixer until the ultramarine is dispersed.
2. Have the fragrance oil to hand. These will be added just prior to pouring the soap into the pan.

Mixing the Soap

1. Slowly pour the lye solution into the large bowl containing the oil mixture. Stir slowly with a wooden spoon. If you prefer, you may stir with the stick mixture with the power off.
2. After all the lye has been added and mixed with the oils, begin to stir with the stick mixer. The oils and sodium hydroxide will start to react to produce soap and glycerin.
3. Continue to stir using the stick mixer. The soap mixture will become more opaque and begin to thicken. You will notice the soap mixture will become more and more like a batter.
4. Add the 30 ml or 2 T ivy fragrance oil to the soap and mix well.
5. Stir until the soap mixture is like a cake batter. At this point the soap will trace, or leave a pattern if drizzled over the surface. The soap is now ready to pour into the soap mould or pan.

Pouring the Soap

1. Once the soap mixture has thickened and is at "trace", it is time to pour the soap mixture into the mould or pan.
2. Slowly pour the soap into the pan. You may use a spatula to scrape the bowl's sides.

3. Gently tilt the pan to distribute the soap mixture until it is even in the pan.
4. Sprinkle the top of the soap with the remainder of the French green clay.
5. Wrap the soap with cling film and cover the soap with layers of towels to keep the heat in.

Soap Processing

1. The soap will continue to process while it is wrapped in the towels. The chemical reaction will continue to produce soap and glycerine from the oil
2. As the chemical reaction occurs and the soap heats further, the soap will enter a "gel" phase. If you peek at the soap you will notice the soap becoming more transparent and darker in the centre. The "gel" spreads to the edge of the pan as the chemical reaction occurs.
3. Once the "gel" has reached the edge, you may unwrap the soap. At this point, there is minimal sodium hydroxide remaining in the soap. You can leave the soap wrapped until it has cooled completely if you prefer.

Finishing the Soap

1. When the soap has cooled, remove the soap from the pan or tray.
2. Cut immediately into pieces. If you wait to cut the soap, it may break when you cut it.
3. Check pH of the finished soap. It will probably be about pH 9. Soap below pH 10 is safe to use.

Oats & Honey Soap

Equipment	Ingredients
Scales	112 g / 4 oz Sodium hydroxide
Rubber gloves	(NaOH)
Large glass jar or a Pyrex measuring cup	200 g / 7 oz Water
Small plastic or glass bowl	150 g / 5.3 oz Olive oil
Large glass bowl	125 g / 4.4 oz Sweet Almond oil
Pan (9x9 inch)	175 g / 6.2 oz Palm oil
Wooden Spoon	468 g / 16.5 oz Coconut oil
Electric stick mixer	15 ml / 1 Dark honey
Microwave oven or bain-marie	2 T Oatmeal
Cling film	15 ml / 1 T Vanilla fragrance oil
Towels	
Measuring spoons, teaspoon, tablespoon	

Making the Lye Solution

Lye Solution	
Water	Sodium Hydroxide (NaOH)
200 grams / 7 oz	112 g / 4 oz
Safety Advice: Always add sodium hydroxide to water!	

1. Gather your gloves and put them on.
2. Place the large glass bowl on the scale and zero the scale to eliminate the weight of the bowl.
3. Weigh the water into the jar so the water weight is 200 g or 7 oz
4. Place the small plastic or glass bowl on the scale and tare out the weight of the bowl or re-zero the scale. Carefully pour the sodium hydroxide into the bowl until you have 112 g or 4 oz of sodium hydroxide.
5. Move to sink and place water jar in the sink. Slowly pour the sodium hydroxide into the large jar containing the water. You can swirl the jar to begin mixing the sodium hydroxide into the water.
6. After you have added all the sodium hydroxide, use the wooden spoon to stir the sodium hydroxide into the water. Ensure all the sodium hydroxide has dissolved into the water. Continue to stir until there are no crystals floating in the solution.
7. Set the lye solution in a safe place and get the oils ready.

Measuring and Mixing the Oils

Oil Mixture			
Olive Oil	Almond Oil	Palm Oil	Coconut Oil
150 grams / 5.3 oz	125 grams / 4.4 oz	175 grams / 6.2 oz	468 grams / 16.5 oz

1. Place the glass bowl on the scale and tare the weight. Weigh 468 g or 16.5 oz of coconut oil into the glass bowl.
2. Zero the scale and weigh the 175 g or 6.2 oz of palm oil into the bowl containing the coconut oil.
3. Transfer the glass bowl with the solid coconut and palm oil to the microwave or bain-marie and heat just until melted.
4. In a large glass bowl, pour the olive oil in until you have 150 g or 5.3 oz.

5. Re-zero the scale and add 125 g or 4.4 oz of the sweet almond oil to the same bowl.

6. Add the melted palm and coconut oil to the larger glass bowl containing the sweet almond and olive oil.

7. Stir all oils together well using either a hand blender or whisk. Your oils are now ready to go.

Additional Ingredients

Additional Ingredients		
Honey	Botanical	Fragrance Oils
Dark	Oatmeal	Vanilla
15 ml or 1 T	2 T	15 ml or 1 T
add to oil mix	add to oil mix	add at trace

1. Add 15 ml or 1 T dark honey and 2 T oatmeal to the oil mixture and stir with the stick mixer.

2. Have the vanilla fragrance oil to hand. This will be added just prior to pouring the soap into the pan.

Mixing the Soap

1. Slowly pour the lye solution into the large bowl containing the oil mixture. Stir slowly with a wooden spoon. If you prefer, you may stir with the stick mixture with the power off.

2. After all the lye has been added and mixed with the oils, begin to stir with the stick mixer. The oils and sodium hydroxide will start to react to produce soap and glycerin.

3. Continue to stir using the stick mixer. The soap mixture will become more opaque and begin to thicken. You will notice the soap mixture will become more and more like a batter.

4. Add the vanilla fragrance oil to the soap mixture and continue to stir.

5. Stir until the soap mixture is like a cake batter. At this point the soap will trace, or leave a pattern if drizzled over the surface. The soap is now ready to pour into the soap mould or pan.

Pouring the Soap

1. Once the soap mixture has thickened and is at "trace", it is time to pour the soap mixture into the mould or pan.
2. Slowly pour the soap into the pan. You may use a spatula to scrape the bowl's sides.
3. Gently tilt the pan to distribute the soap mixture until it is even in the pan.
4. Wrap the soap with cling film and cover the soap with layers of towels to keep the heat in.

Soap Processing

1. The soap will continue to process while it is wrapped in the towels. The chemical reaction will continue to produce soap and glycerine from the oil
2. As the chemical reaction occurs and the soap heats further, the soap will enter a "gel" phase. If you peek at the soap you will notice the soap becoming more transparent and darker in the centre. The "gel" spreads to the edge of the pan as the chemical reaction occurs.
3. Once the "gel" has reached the edge, you may unwrap the soap. At this point, there is minimal sodium hydroxide remaining in the soap. You can leave the soap wrapped until it has cooled completely if you prefer.

Finishing the Soap

1. When the soap has cooled, remove the soap from the pan or tray.
2. Cut immediately into pieces. If you wait to cut the soap, it may break when you cut it.
3. Check pH of the finished soap. It will probably be about pH 9. Soap below pH 10 is safe to use.

Nut & Honey Soap

Equipment	*Ingredients*
Scales	125 g / 4.4 oz Sodium hydroxide
Rubber gloves	(NaOH)
Large glass jar or a Pyrex measuring cup	225 g / 7.9 oz Water
Small plastic or glass bowl	300 g / 10.6 oz Hazelnut oil
Large glass bowl	200 g / 7.1 oz Peanut oil
Pan (9x9 inch)	500 g / 17.6 oz Palm oil
Wooden Spoon	15 ml / 1 T Heather honey
Electric Stick Mixer	30 ml/ 2 T Almond fragrance oil
Microwave oven or bain-Marie	½ tsp Cinnamon powder
Cling film	
Towels	
Measuring spoons, teaspoon, tablespoon	

Making the Lye Solution

Lye Solution	
Water	Sodium Hydroxide (NaOH)
225 grams / 7.9 oz	125 g / 4.4 oz
Safety Advice: Always add sodium hydroxide to water!	

1. Put on your gloves before you begin
2. Place the large glass jar on the scale and re-zero the scale to eliminate the weight of the jar.
3. Weigh the water into the jar so the water weight is 225 g or 7.9 ounces.
4. Place the small plastic or glass bowl on the scale and tare out the weight of the bowl or re-zero the scale. Carefully pour the sodium hydroxide into the bowl until you have 125 g or 4.4 oz of sodium hydroxide.
5. Move to sink and place water jar in the sink. Slowly pour the sodium hydroxide into the large jar containing the water. You can swirl the jar to begin mixing the sodium hydroxide into the water.
6. After you have added all the sodium hydroxide, use the wooden spoon to stir the sodium hydroxide. Ensure all the sodium hydroxide has dissolved into the water. Continue to stir until there are no crystals floating in the solution.
7. Set the lye solution in a safe place and get the oils ready.

Measuring and Mixing the Oils

Oil Mixture		
Hazelnut Oil	Peanut Oil	Palm Oil
300 grams / 10.6 oz	200 grams / 7.1 oz	500 grams / 17.6 oz

1. Place the glass bowl on the scale. Zero the scale and weigh 500 g or 17.6 oz of palm oil into the glass bowl.
2. Transfer the glass bowl with the solid palm oil to the microwave or bain-marie and heat just until melted.
3. In a large glass bowl, pour the hazelnut oil in until you have 300 g or 10.6 oz.
4. Re-zero the scale and add 200 g or 7.1 oz of the peanut oil to the same bowl.
5. Add the melted palm to the larger glass bowl containing the hazelnut and peanut oil.
6. Stir all oils together well using either a hand blender or spoon. Your oils are now ready to go.

Additional Ingredients

Additional Ingredients		
Honey	Spice	Fragrance Oil
Heather 15 ml or 1 T	Cinnamon ½ tsp	Almond 30 ml or 2 T
add to oil mix	add to oil mix	add at trace

1. Add 15 ml or 1 T heather honey into to the oil mixture and stir.
2. Add to ½ tsp cinnamon to the oil mixture. Stir.
3. Have the almond fragrance oil to hand.

Mixing the Soap

1. Slowly pour the lye solution into the large bowl containing the oil mixture. Stir slowly with a wooden spoon. If you prefer, you may stir with the stick mixture with the power off.

2. After all the lye has been added and mixed with the oils, begin to stir with the stick mixer. The oils and sodium hydroxide will start to react to produce soap and glycerin.
3. Continue to stir using the stick mixer. The soap mixture will become more opaque and begin to thicken. You will notice the soap mixture will become more and more like a batter.
4. Add the almond fragrance oil to the soap mixture and continue to stir.
5. Stir until the soap mixture is like a cake batter. At this point the soap will trace, or leave a pattern if drizzled over the surface. The soap is now ready to pour into the soap mould or pan.

Pouring the Soap

1. Once the soap mixture has thickened and is at "trace", it is time to pour the soap mixture into the mould or pan.
2. Slowly pour the soap into the pan. You may use a spatula to scrape the bowl's sides.
3. Gently tilt the pan to distribute the soap mixture until it is even in the pan.
4. Wrap the soap with cling film and cover the soap with layers of towels to keep the heat in.

Soap Processing

1. The soap will continue to process while it is wrapped in the towels. The chemical reaction will continue to produce soap and glycerine from the oil
2. As the chemical reaction occurs and the soap heats further, the soap will enter a "gel" phase. If you peek at the soap you will notice the soap becoming more transparent and darker in the centre. The "gel" spreads to the edge of the pan as the chemical reaction occurs.
3. Once the "gel" has reached the edge, you may unwrap the soap. At this point, there is minimal sodium hydroxide remaining in the soap. You can leave the soap wrapped until it has cooled completely if you prefer.

Finishing the Soap

1. When the soap has cooled, remove the soap from the pan or tray.
2. Cut immediately into pieces. If you wait to cut the soap, it may break when you cut it.
3. Check pH of the finished soap. It will probably be about pH 9. Soap is below pH 10 it is safe to use.

Blue Moon Honey Soap

Equipment
Scales
Rubber gloves
Large glass jar or a Pyrex measuring cup
Small plastic or glass bowl
Large glass bowl
Pan (9x9 inch)
Wooden spoon
Electric sick mixer
Microwave oven or bain-marie
Cling film
Towels

Ingredients
120 g / 4.2 oz Sodium hydroxide (NaOH)
215 g / 7.6 oz Water
300 g / 10.6 oz Olive oil
200 g / 7.1 oz Sweet almond oil
450 g / 15.9 oz Vegetable shortening
15 ml / 1 T Lavender honey
¼ tsp Ultramarine blue
1 T Blue poppy seeds
30 ml/ 2 T Blackberry sage fragrance oil

Making the Lye Solution

Lye Solution	
Water	Sodium Hydroxide (NaOH)
215 grams / 7.6 oz	120 g / 4.2 oz
Safety Advice: Always add sodium hydroxide to water!	

1. Before you begin, put on your gloves.
2. Place the large glass jar on the scale. Zero the scale.
3. Weigh the water into the jar so the water weight is 215 g or 7.6 oz.
4. Place the small plastic or glass bowl on the scale, zero the scale and carefully pour the sodium hydroxide into the bowl until you have 120 g or 4.2 oz of sodium hydroxide.
5. Move to sink and place water jar in the sink. Slowly pour the sodium hydroxide into the large jar containing the water. You can swirl the jar to begin mixing the sodium hydroxide into the water.
6. After you have added all the sodium hydroxide, use the wooden spoon to stir the sodium hydroxide. Ensure all the sodium hydroxide has dissolved into the water. Continue to stir until there are no crystals floating in the solution.
7. Set the lye solution in a safe place and get the oils ready.

Measuring and Mixing the Oils

Oil Mixture		
Olive Oil	Sweet Almond Oil	Veg,. Shortening
300 grams / 10.6 oz	200 grams / 7.1 oz	450 grams / 15.9 oz

1. Place the glass bowl on the scale and zero the scale. Weigh 450 g or 15.9 oz of vegetable shortening into the glass bowl.
2. Transfer the glass bowl with the solid vegetable shortening to the microwave or bain-marie and heat just until melted.
3. In a large glass bowl, pour the olive oil in until you have 300 g or 10.6 oz.
4. Re-zero the scale and add 200 g or 7.1 oz of the sweet almond oil to the same bowl.
5. Add the melted vegetable shortening to the larger glass bowl containing the olive oil and sweet almond oil.
6. Stir all oils together well using either a hand blender or spoon. Your oils are now ready to go.

Additional Ingredients

Additional Ingredients			
Honey	Colour	Botanical	Fragrance Oils
Lavender	Ultramarine Blue	Poppy seeds	Blackberry Sage
15 ml or 1 T	¼ tsp	1T	30 ml or 2 T
add to oil mix	add to oil mix	add to oil mix	add at trace

1. Add 15 ml or 1 T lavender honey to to the oil mixture and stir.
2. Add ¼ tsp ultramarine blue to the oil mixture. Stir with the stick mixture until the ultramarine blue is dispersed.
3. Add 1T blue poppy seeds to the oil mixture. These look like little moon rocks!
4. Have the blackberry sage fragrance oil to hand.

Mixing the Soap

1. Slowly pour the lye solution into the large bowl containing the oil mixture. Stir slowly with a wooden spoon. If you prefer, you may stir with the stick mixture with the power off.
2. After all the lye has been added and mixed with the oils, begin to stir with the stick mixer on. The oils and sodium hydroxide will start to react to produce soap and glycerin.
3. Continue to stir using the stick mixer. The soap mixture will become more opaque and begin to thicken. You will notice the soap mixture will become more and more like a batter.
4. Add the blackberry sage fragrance oil to the soap mixture and continue to stir.
5. Stir until the soap mixture is like a cake batter. At this point the soap will trace, or leave a pattern if drizzled over the surface. The soap is now ready to pour into the soap mould or pan.

Pouring the Soap

1. Once the soap mixture has thickened and is at "trace", it is time to pour the soap mixture into the mould or pan.
2. Slowly pour the soap into the pan. You may use a spatula to scrape the bowl's sides.
3. Gently tilt the pan to distribute the soap mixture until it is even in the pan.
4. Wrap the soap with cling film and cover the soap with layers of towels to keep the heat in.

Soap Processing

1. The soap will continue to process while it is wrapped in the towels. The chemical reaction will continue to produce soap and glycerine from the oil
2. As the chemical reaction occurs and the soap heats further, the soap will enter a "gel" phase. If you peek at the soap you will notice the soap becoming more transparent and darker in the centre. The "gel" spreads to the edge of the pan as the chemical reaction occurs.
3. Once the "gel" has reached the edge, you may unwrap the soap. At this point, there is minimal sodium hydroxide remaining in the soap. You can leave the soap wrapped until it has cooled completely if you prefer.

Finishing the Soap

1. When the soap has cooled, remove the soap from the pan or tray.
2. Cut immediately into pieces. If you wait to cut the soap, it may break when you cut it.
3. Check pH of the finished soap. It will probably be about pH 9. Soap below pH 10 is safe to use.

Sunny Honey Soap

Equipment	*Ingredients*
Scales	125 g / 4.4 oz Sodium hydroxide
Rubber gloves	(NaOH)
Large glass jar or a Pyrex measuring cup	225 g / 7.9 oz Water
Small plastic or glass bowl	300 g / 10.6 oz Olive oil
Large glass bowl	200 g / 7.1 oz Sunflower oil
Pan (9x9 inch)	500 g / 17.6 oz Palm oil
Wooden spoon	1/8 tsp Yellow iron oxide
Electric stick mixer	15 ml / 1 T Sunflower honey
Microwave oven or bain-marie	30 ml /2 T Sunflower fragrance oil
Cling film	
Towels	

Making the Lye Solution

Lye Solution	
Water	**Sodium Hydroxide (NaOH)**
225 grams / 7.9 oz	125 g / 4.4 oz
Safety Advice: Always add sodium hydroxide to water!	

1. Put on your gloves before you begin.
2. Place the large glass jar on the scale and zero the scale.
3. Weigh the water into the jar so the water weight is 225 g or 7.9 oz.
4. Place the small plastic or glass bowl on the scale and tare out the weight of the bowl or re-zero the scale. Carefully pour the sodium hydroxide into the bowl until you have 125 g or 4.4 oz of sodium hydroxide.
5. Move to sink and place water jar in the sink. Slowly pour the sodium hydroxide into the large jar containing the water. You can swirl the jar to begin mixing the sodium hydroxide into the water.

6. After you have added all the sodium hydroxide, use the wooden spoon to stir the sodium hydroxide. Continue to stir until there are no crystals floating in the solution.
7. Set the lye solution in a safe place and get the oils ready.

Measuring and Mixing the Oils

Oil Mixture		
Olive Oil	Sunflower Oil	Palm Oil
300 grams / 10.6 oz	200 grams / 7.1 oz	500 grams / 17.6 oz

1. Place the glass bowl on the scale and zero the scale. Weigh 500 g or 17.6 oz of palm oil into the glass bowl.
2. Transfer the glass bowl with the solid palm oil to the microwave or Bain-marie and heat just until melted.
3. In a large glass bowl, pour the olive oil in until you have 300 g or 10.6 oz.
4. Zero the scale and add 200 g or 7.1 oz of the sunflower oil to the same bowl.
5. Add the melted palm oil to the larger glass bowl containing the sunflower and olive oil.
6. Stir all oils together well using either a hand blender or whisk. Your oils are now ready to go.

Additional Ingredients

Additional Ingredients		
Honey	Colour	Fragrance Oil
Sunflower	Yellow Iron Oxide	Sunflower
15 ml or 1 T	$1/8$ tsp	30 ml or 2 T
add to oil mix	add to oil mix	add at trace

1. Add 15 ml or 1 T sunflower honey into to the oil mixture and stir.
2. Add $1/8$ tsp yellow iron oxide to the oil mixture. Stir until all the yellow oxide is dispersed in the oil and honey mixture.
3. Have the sunflower fragrance oil to hand.

Mixing the Soap

1. Slowly pour the lye solution into the large bowl containing the oil mixture. Stir slowly with a wooden spoon. If you prefer, you may stir with the stick mixture with the power off.
2. After all the lye has been added and mixed with the oils, begin to stir with the stick mixer. The oils and sodium hydroxide will start to react to produce soap and glycerin.
3. Continue to stir using the stick mixer. The soap mixture will become more opaque and begin to thicken. You will notice the soap mixture will become more and more like a batter.
4. Add the sunflower fragrance oil to the soap mixture and continue to stir.
5. Stir until the soap mixture is like a cake batter. At this point the soap will trace, or leave a pattern if drizzled over the surface. The soap is now ready to pour into the soap mould or pan.

Pouring the Soap

1. Once the soap mixture has thickened and is at "trace", it is time to pour the soap mixture into the mould or pan.
2. Slowly pour the soap into the pan. You may use a spatula to scrape the sides.
3. Gently tilt the pan to distribute the soap mixture until it is even in the pan.
4. Wrap the soap with cling film and cover the soap with layers of towels to keep the heat in.

Soap Processing

1. The soap will continue to process while it is wrapped in the towels. The chemical reaction will continue to produce soap and glycerine from the oil
2. As the chemical reaction occurs and the soap heats further, the soap will enter a "gel" phase. If you peek at the soap you will notice the soap becoming more transparent and darker in the centre. The "gel" spreads to the edge of the pan as the chemical reaction occurs.
3. Once the "gel" has reached the edge, you may unwrap the soap. At this point, there is minimal sodium hydroxide remaining in the soap. You can leave the soap wrapped until it has cooled completely if you prefer.

Finishing the Soap

1. When the soap has cooled, remove the soap from the pan or tray.
2. Cut immediately into pieces. If you wait to cut the soap, it may break when you cut it.
3. Check pH of the finished soap. It will probably be about pH 9. Soap below pH 10 is safe to use.

Rose Hip & Honey Soap

Equipment
Scales
Rubber gloves
Large glass jar or a Pyrex measuring cup
Small plastic or glass bowl
Large glass bowl
Pan (9x9 inch)
Wooden spoon
Electric stick mixer
Microwave oven or bain-marie
Cling film
Towels
Measuring spoons, teaspoon, tablespoon

Ingredients
103 g / 3.6 oz Sodium hydroxide (NaOH)
190 g / 6.7 oz Water
200 g / 7.1 oz Olive oil
200 g / 7.1 oz Coconut oil
400 g / 14 oz   Palm oil
1 Sachet/ 1 T Rose hip tea
15 ml / 1 T Blossom honey
30 ml/ 2 T Rose fragrance oil

Making the Lye Solution

Lye Solution	
Water	Sodium Hydroxide (NaOH)
190 g / 6.7 oz	103 g / 3.6 oz
Safety Advice: Always add sodium hydroxide to water!	

1. Put on your gloves.
2. Place the large glass jar on the scale and zero the scale .
3. Weigh the water into the jar so the water weight is 190 g or 6.7 oz.
4. Place the small plastic or glass bowl on the scale and re-zero the scale. Carefully pour the sodium hydroxide into the bowl until you have 103 g or 3.6 oz of sodium hydroxide.

5. Move to sink and place water jar in the sink. Slowly pour the sodium hydroxide into the large jar containing the water. You can swirl the jar to begin mixing the sodium hydroxide into the water.

6. After you have added all the sodium hydroxide, use the wooden spoon to stir the sodium hydroxide. Continue to stir until there are no crystals floating in the solution.

7. Set the lye solution in a safe place and get the oils ready.

Measuring and Mixing the Oils

Oil Mixture		
Olive Oil	Coconut Oil	Palm Oil
200 grams / 7.1 oz	200 grams / 7.1 oz	400 grams / 14 oz

1. Place the glass bowl on the scale and zero the scale. Weigh 400 g or 14 oz of palm oil into the glass bowl.

2. Re-zero the scale and weigh the 200 g or 7.1 oz of coconut oil into the bowl containing the palm oil.

3. Transfer the glass bowl with the solid coconut and palm oil to the microwave or Bain-marie and heat just until melted.

4. In a large glass bowl, pour the olive oil in until you have 200 g or 7.1 oz.

5. Add the melted palm and coconut oil to the larger glass bowl containing the olive oil.

6. Stir all oils together well using either a hand blender or spoon. Your oils are now ready to go.

Additional Ingredients

Additional Ingredients		
Honey	Botanical	Fragrance Oil
Blossom	Rose Hip Tea	Rose
15 ml or 1 T	1 sachet or 1 T	30 ml or 2 T
add to oil mix	add to oil mix	add at trace

1. Add 15 ml or 1 T blossom honey into to the oil mixture and stir.
2. Add the contents of 1 sachet rose hip tea to the oil mixture. Stir.
3. Have the rose fragrance oil to hand.

Mixing the Soap

1. Slowly pour the lye solution into the large bowl containing the oil mixture. Stir slowly with a wooden spoon. If you prefer, you may stir with the stick mixture with the power off.
2. After all the lye has been added and mixed with the oils, begin to stir with the stick mixer. The oils and sodium hydroxide will start to react to produce soap and glycerin.
3. Continue to stir using the stick mixer on. The soap mixture will become more opaque and begin to thicken. You will notice the soap mixture will become more and more like a batter.
4. Add the rose fragrance oil to the soap mixture and continue to stir.

Pouring the Soap

1. Once the soap mixture has thickened and is at "trace", it is time to pour the soap mixture into the mould or pan.
2. Slowly pour the soap into the pan. You may use a spatula to scrape the sides.
3. Gently tilt the pan to distribute the soap mixture until it is even in the pan.
4. Wrap the soap with cling film and cover the soap with layers of towels to keep the heat in.

Soap Processing

1. The soap will continue to process while it is wrapped in the towels. The chemical reaction will continue to produce soap and glycerine from the oil
2. As the chemical reaction occurs and the soap heats further, the soap will enter a "gel" phase. If you peek at the soap you will notice the soap becoming more transparent and darker in the centre. The "gel" spreads to the edge of the pan as the chemical reaction occurs.
3. Once the "gel" has reached the edge, you may unwrap the soap. At this point, there is minimal sodium hydroxide remaining in the soap. You can leave the soap wrapped until it has cooled completely if you prefer.

Finishing the Soap

1. When the soap has cooled, remove the soap from the pan or tray.
2. Cut immediately into pieces. If you wait to cut the soap, it may break when you cut it.
3. Check pH of the finished soap. It will probably be about pH 9. Soap below pH 10 is safe to use.

Avocado Spa Soap

Equipment	*Ingredients*
Scales	112 g / 4 oz Sodium hydroxide
Rubber gloves	(NaOH)
Large glass jar or a Pyrex measuring cup	200 g / 7 oz Water
Small plastic or glass bowl	150 g / 5.3 oz Olive oil
Large glass bowl	125 g / 4.4 oz Avocado oil
Pan (9x9 inch)	175 g / 6.2 oz Palm oil
Wooden spoon	468 g / 16.5 oz Coconut oil
Electric stick mixer	1/8 tsp Chromium green oxide
Microwave oven or bain-marie	15 ml / 1 T Dark honey
Cling film	30 ml/ 2 T Rosemary fragrance oil
Towels	
Measuring spoons, teaspoon, tablespoon	

Making the Lye Solution

Lye Solution	
Water	Sodium Hydroxide (NaOH)
200 grams / 7 oz	112 g / 4 oz
Safety Advice: Always add sodium hydroxide to water!	

1. Before you begin, put on your gloves.
2. Place the large glass jar on the scale and zero the scale to eliminate the weight of the jar.
3. Weigh the water into the jar so the water weight is 200 g or 7 ounces.
4. Place the small plastic or glass bowl on the scale and zero the scale. Carefully pour the sodium hydroxide into the bowl until you have 112 g or 4 oz of sodium hydroxide.

5. Move to sink and place water jar in the sink. Slowly pour the sodium hydroxide into the large jar containing the water. You can swirl the jar to begin mixing the sodium hydroxide into the water.
6. After you have added all the sodium hydroxide, use the wooden spoon to stir the sodium hydroxide. Ensure all the sodium hydroxide has dissolved into the water. Continue to stir until there are no crystals floating in the solution.
7. Set the lye solution in a safe place and get the oils ready.

Measuring and Mixing the Oils

Oil Mixture			
Olive Oil	Advocado Oil	Palm Oil	Coconut Oil
150 grams / 5.3 oz	125 grams / 4.4 oz	175 grams / 6.2 oz	468 grams / 16.5 oz

1. Place the glass bowl on the scale and tare the weight, or re-zero the scale. Weigh 468 g or 16.5 oz of coconut oil into the glass bowl.
2. Re-zero the scale and weigh the 175 g or 6.2 oz of palm oil into the bowl containing the coconut oil.
3. Transfer the glass bowl with the solid coconut and palm oil to the microwave or bain-marie and heat just until melted.
4. In a large glass bowl, pour the olive oil in until you have 150 g or 5.3 oz.
5. Re-zero the scale and add 125 g or 4.4 oz of the avocado oil to the same bowl.
6. Add the melted palm and coconut oil to the larger glass bowl containing the avocado and olive oil.
7. Stir all oils together well using either a hand blender or whisk. Your oils are now ready to go.

Additional Ingredients

Additional Ingredients		
Honey	Colour	Fragrance Oils
Dark	Chromium Green Oxide	Rosemary
15 ml / 1T	1/8 tsp	30 ml / 2 T
add to oil mix	add to oil mix	add at trace

1. Add 15 ml or 1 T dark honey and 1/8 tsp chromium green oxide to the oil mixture and stir with the stick mixer until the chromium green oxide is dispersed.
2. Have the rosemary fragrance oil to hand. This will be added just prior to pouring the soap into the pan.

Mixing the Soap

1. Slowly pour the lye solution into the large bowl containing the oil mixture. Stir slowly with a wooden spoon. If you prefer, you may stir with the stick mixture with the power off.
2. After all the lye has been added and mixed with the oils, begin to stir with the stick mixer on. The oils and sodium hydroxide will start to react to produce soap and glycerin.
3. Continue to stir using the stick mixer. The soap mixture will become more opaque and begin to thicken. You will notice the soap mixture will become more and more like a batter.
4. Add the rosemary fragrance oil to the soap mixture and continue to stir.
5. Stir until the soap mixture is like a cake batter. At this point the soap will trace, or leave a pattern if drizzled over the surface. The soap is now ready to pour into the soap mould or pan.

Pouring the Soap

1. Once the soap mixture has thickened and is at "trace", it is time to pour the soap mixture into the mould or pan.
2. Slowly pour the soap into the pan. You may use a spatula to scrape the bowl's sides.
3. Gently tilt the pan to distribute the soap mixture until it is even in the pan.
4. Wrap the soap with cling film and cover the soap with layers of towels to keep the heat in.

Soap Processing

4. The soap will continue to process while it is wrapped in the towels. The chemical reaction will continue to produce soap and glycerine from the oil
5. As the chemical reaction occurs and the soap heats further, the soap will enter a "gel" phase. If you peek at the soap you will notice the soap becoming more transparent and darker in the centre. The "gel" spreads to the edge of the pan as the chemical reaction occurs.
6. Once the "gel" has reached the edge, you may unwrap the soap. At this point,

there is minimal sodium hydroxide remaining in the soap. You can leave the soap wrapped until it has cooled completely if you prefer

Finishing the Soap

4. When the soap has cooled, remove the soap from the pan or tray.
5. Cut immediately into pieces. If you wait to cut the soap, it may break when you cut it.
6. Check pH of the finished soap. It will probably be about pH 9. Soap below pH 10 is safe to use.

Oil	SAP	KOH Factor	NaOH Factor
Almond Oil	193	0.193	0.137
Apricot Kernel Oil	192	0.192	0.137
Avocado Oil	188	0.188	0.134
Babassu Nut Oil	246	0.246	0.176
Beeswax	96	0.096	0.068
Borage Oil	189	0.189	0.134
Candelilla Wax	52	0.052	0.037
Canola Oil	187	0.187	0.133
Castor Oil	181	0.181	0.129
Cherry Kernel Oil	196	0.196	0.139
Cocoa Butter	192	0.192	0.137
Coconut Oil	258	0.258	0.184
Corn Oil	193	0.193	0.137
Cottonseed Oil	195	0.195	0.139
Vegetable Shortening	193	0.193	0.137
Flaxseed Oil	191	0.191	0.136
Grapeseed Oil	186	0.186	0.133
Hazelnut Oil	193	0.193	0.137
Hempseed Oil	191	0.191	0.136
Jojoba Seed Oil	94	0.094	0.067
Karite Butter (Shea Butter)	183	0.183	0.130
Kukui Nut Oil	190	0.190	0.136
Lanolin	105	0.105	0.075
Lard	197	0.197	0.140
Linseed Oil	191	0.191	0.136
Macadamia Nut Oil	196	0.196	0.140
Mango Butter	186	0.186	0.133
Neem Tree Oil	194	0.194	0.141
Olive Oil	191	0.191	0.136
Palm Kernel Oil	240	0.240	0.171
Palm Oil	200	0.200	0.143
Peach Kernel Oil	192	0.192	0.137
Peanut Oil	193	0.193	0.137
Pumpkin Seed Oil	196	0.196	0.139
Rapeseed Oil	187	0.187	0.133
Rice Bran Oil	181	0.181	0.129
Safflower Oil	194	0.194	0.138
Sesame Seed Oil	188	0.188	0.134
Soybean Oil	191	0.191	0.136
Sunflower Seed Oil	191	0.191	0.136
Tallow, Beef	200	0.200	0.142
Walnut Oil	190	0.190	0.135
Wheat Germ Oil	186	0.186	0.132

INCI	Potassium Soap	Sodium Soap
Prunus Amygdalus Dulcis	Potassium Almondate	Sodium Almondate
Prunus Armeniaca Kernel	PotassiumApricot Kernelate	Sodium Apricot Kernelate
Persea Gratissima	Potassium Avocadate	Sodium Avocadate
Orbignya Oleifera	Potassium Babassuate	Sodium Babassuate
Beeswax	Potassium Beeswax	Sodium Beeswax
Borago Officinalis	Potassium Boragate	Sodium Boragate
Euphorbia Cerifera	Potassium Candelillate	Sodium Candelillate
Canola Oil	Potassium Canolate	Sodium Canolate
Ricinus Communis	Potassium Castorate	Sodium Castorate
Prunus avium	Potassium Cherry Kernelate	Sodium Cherry Kernelate
Theobroma Cacao	Potassium Cocoa Butterate	Sodium Cocoa Butterate
Cocos Nucifera	Potassium Cocoate	Sodium Cocoate
Zea Mays Oil	Potassium Cornate	Sodium Cornate
Gossypium Barbadense	Potassium Cottonseedate	Sodium Cottonseedate
Vegetable Shortening	*	*
Linum Usitatissimum	Potassium Flaxseedate	Sodium Flaxseedate
Vitis Vinifera	Potassium Grapeseedate	Sodium Grapeseedate
Corylus Americana	Potassium Hazel Seedate	Sodium Hazel Seedate
Cannabis Sativa	Potassium Hemp Seedate	Sodium Hemp Seedate
Simmondsia Chinensis	Potassium Jojoba Seedate	Sodium Jojoba Seedate
Butyrospermum Parkii	Potassium Shea Butterate	Sodium Shea Butterate
Aleurites Molaccana	Potassium Kukui Seedate	Sodium Kukui Seedate
Lanolin	Potassium Lanolinate	Sodium Lanolinate
Lard	Potassium Lardate	Sodium Lardate
Linum Usitatissmum	Potassium Linseedate	Sodium Linseedate
Macadamia Ternifolia	Potassium Macadamia Seedate	Sodium Macadamia Seedate
Mangifera Indica	Potassium Mango Butterate	Sodium Mango Butterate
Melia Azadirachta	Potassium Neemate	Sodium Neemate
Olea europaea	Potassium Olivate	Sodium Olivate
Elaeis Guineensis	Potassium Palm Kernelate	Sodium Palm Kernelate
Elaeis Guineensis	Potassium Palmate	Sodium Palmate
Prunus Persica	Potassium Peach Kernelate	Sodium Peach Kernelate
Arachis Hypogaea	Potassium Peanutate	Sodium Peanutate
Cucurbita Pepo	Potassium Pumpkin Seedate	Sodium Pumpkin Seedate
Brassica Campestris	Potassium Rapeseedate	Sodium Rapeseedate
Oryza Sativa	Potassium Rice Branate	Sodium Rice Branate
Carthamus Tinctorius	Potassium Safflowerate	Sodium Safflowerate
Sesamum Indicum	Potassium Sesame Seedate	Sodium Sesame Seedate
Glycine Soja	Potassium Soybeanate	Sodium Soybeanate
Helianthus Annuus	Potassium Sunflower Seedate	Sodium Sunflower Seedate
Tallow	Potassium Tallowate	Sodium Tallowate
Juglans Regia	Potassium Walnutate	Sodium Walnutate
Tritium Vulgare	Potassium Wheat Germate	Sodium Wheat Germate

* varies by oils used in shortening

Oil	Weight		NaOH Factor		NaOH
Almond Oil	X		0.137	=	
Apricot Kernel Oil	X		0.137	=	
Avocado Oil	X		0.134	=	
Babassu Nut Oil	X		0.176	=	
Beeswax	X		0.068	=	
Borage Oil	X		0.134	=	
Candelilla Wax	X		0.037	=	
Canola Oil	X		0.133	=	
Castor Oil	X		0.129	=	
Cherry Kernel Oil	X		0.139	=	
Cocoa Butter	X		0.137	=	
Coconut Oil	X		0.184	=	
Corn Oil	X		0.137	=	
Cottonseed Oil	X		0.139	=	
Vegetable Shortening	X		0.137	=	
Flaxseed Oil	X		0.136	=	
Grapeseed Oil	X		0.133	=	
Hazelnut Oil	X		0.137	=	
Hempseed Oil	X		0.136	=	
Jojoba Seed Oil	X		0.067	=	
Karite Butter (Shea Butter)	X		0.130	=	
Kukui Nut Oil	X		0.136	=	
Lanolin	X		0.075	=	
Lard	X		0.140	=	
Linseed Oil	X		0.136	=	
Macadamia Nut Oil	X		0.140	=	
Mango Butter	X		0.133	=	
Neem Tree Oil	X		0.141	=	
Olive Oil	X		0.136	=	
Palm Kernel Oil	X		0.171	=	
Palm Oil	X		0.143	=	
Peach Kernel Oil	X		0.137	=	
Peanut Oil	X		0.137	=	
Pumpkin Seed Oil	X		0.139	=	
Rapeseed Oil	X		0.133	=	
Rice Bran Oil	X		0.129	=	
Safflower Oil	X		0.138	=	
Sesame Seed Oil	X		0.134	=	
Soybean Oil	X		0.136	=	
Sunflower Seed Oil	X		0.136	=	
Tallow, Beef	X		0.142	=	
Walnut Oil	X		0.135	=	
Wheat Germ Oil	X		0.132	=	
			Total	=	

Do not use this amount! Carry the total weight of the NaOH to the table below.

1. Design Your Recipe

Put the weight for each oil in the weight column. You can use either grams or ounces but you must use only one unit for each formulation. In other words, all the values you put in the table above must be in only one unit and all subsequent values used in the other tables in the same units. Multiply by the NaOH Factor. Total the values in the NaOH column.

2. Calculate the amount of NaOH

Superfatting	Factor	Above NaOH	NaOH to use
For 6% Superfatted	0.94	X	=
For 10% Superfatted	0.90	X	=
For 15% Superfatted	0.85	X	=

Carry the total calculated NaOH amount from the above table to the supperfatting table below. Put the total NaOH in the column labelled "above NaOH". Multiply the above value by the supperfatting factor. This gives you the amount of NaOH to use in your recipe.

3. Determine the amount of Water

Lye Solution	NaOH	Water Factor	Water to Use
For 30% w/w	÷	0.43	=
For 33% w/w	÷	0.49	=
For 36% w/w	÷	0.56	=

After you have determined the amount of NaOH to use in your recipe, you need to determine how much water you need to make your lye solution. The higher the concentration of the solution, the faster the oils will saponify and the soap will reach a safe pH.

Note: w/w % solution is calculated as follows

Weight of solute/ (weight of solute + weight of solvent) × 100

Example:
112 g NaOH / (112 g NaOH + 200 g water) × 100=
112 g/312 g × 100=
.36 × 100= 36% w/w

A note about suppliers

When I began to make soap I was at a loss as to where to get the equipment and ingredients needed. I am sure many of you are wondering the same thing. I considered adding a supplier list to the back of Dr Sara's Honey Potions. I decided against this because one of the aims of my book is to provide you with recipes you can make with items available to you at local shops and without specialist equipment. Many of the recipes fall into this category. There are some recipes included in my book which use ingredients which are more specialised. Most of these can be found with ease on the internet. There are internet suppliers for cosmetic containers, fragrances and specialty oils.

The ingredients which can be found most easily include the oils used in soapmaking, such as olive and sunflower. These can be purchased from your grocery store. Coconut oil may be purchased in Asian shops. Palm oil may be a little more difficult to find. Asian food stores will likely have the unrefined palm oil. This is an orange colour and is used in the same way as the refined palm oil. Refined palm oil is used in bakeries and other fast food restaurants as frying oil. Perhaps they would be willing to sell you some or suggest a supplier. Sodium hydroxide (caustic soda) is available in chemists and hardware shops in the UK. Make sure the purity is 98% to ensure the sodium hydroxide will be of the appropriate concentration in the soap recipes. In the US, sodium hydroxide is more difficult to obtain. There are internet sites which sell sodium hydroxide for soapmaking.

Lip balms can made with a number of unusual cosmetic oils and butters. These are best purchased online unless you are lucky enough to have a craft shop nearby which sells these ingredients. Simply search for cocoa, mango or shea butter and you will find a number of suppliers. Cocoa butter will likely be the easiest to find so you may wish to start with a lip balm recipe using cocoa butter.

Recipes for bath bombs begin with two main ingredients, sodium bicarbonate and citric acid. If you are interested in making a small batch of bath bombs, then you should start with your local grocery shop. Most grocery stores will at least stock bicarbonate of soda and many may have citric acid. If your shop does not sell citric acid, you may find it at an Asian food store. When buying larger quantities of sodium bicarbonate and citric acid, a craft shop or online supplier will give you a better price. The colours used in bath bombs can be food colouring or specialist cosmetic colorants. Most of us have food colouring in our kitchen cupboards which we purchased at the grocery store. Food colouring is an inexpensive way to colour your bath bombs. Alternatively, if you would like to try using cosmetic colours, these are available at craft shops or online shops.

Base cosmetics, cosmetic containers, colour pigments, fragrances and flavouring tend to be sold in craft shops, soapmaking shops or by cosmetic supply companies. As making cosmetics becomes more popular the supplies available in craft stores become more varied. You will very likely find a good selection of ingredients and containers in a local craft shop. Essential oils can also be found in many chemists or pharmacies. They may be a little more expensive than in a craft shop but if you do not have a craft store nearby, then you may be willing to pay a little extra. For those of you who do not have a craft supply shop at your convenience, again, look for these items on the internet.

I suggest you start with recipes that use ingredients you can buy at local shops. If you enjoy making Dr Sara's Honey Potions, then move on to the recipes which use more specialist ingredients.
Dr Sara

To contact Dr Sara:

Dr Sara Robb
Bath Potions Ltd
14 Grand Arcade
London, N12 0EH
+44 (0)208 446 6446
sara@bathpotions.com
www.bathpotions.com

Lightning Source UK Ltd.
Milton Keynes UK
UKOW021055130313

207573UK00003B/39/P